Simplified
Interpretation of
ICD Electrograms

For Heather, A.J., and . . .

Simplified Interpretation of ICD Electrograms

Aaron B. Hesselson, MD, BSE, FACC
Assistant Clinical Professor of Medicine
Wayne State University School of Medicine, Detroit, MI

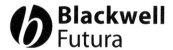

© 2005 by Blackwell Publishing
Blackwell Futura is an imprint of Blackwell Publishing

Blackwell Publishing, Inc., 350 Main Street, Malden, Massachusetts 02148-5020, USA
Blackwell Publishing Ltd, 9600 Garsington Road, Oxford OX4 2DQ, UK
Blackwell Science Asia Pty Ltd, 550 Swanston Street, Carlton, Victoria 3053, Australia

First published 2005
2   2006

ISBN-13: 978-1-4051-2731-8
ISBN-10: 1-4051-2731-7

Library of Congress Cataloging-in-Publication Data

Hesselson, Aaron B.
  Simplified interpretation of ICD electrograms / Aaron B. Hesselson.
    p. ; cm.
  Companion v. to: Simplified interpretation of pacemaker ECGs / Aaron
B. Hesselson. c2003.
  Includes bibliographical references and index.
  ISBN-13: 978-1-4051-2731-8
  ISBN-10: 1-4051-2731-7
  1. Implantable cardioverter-defibrillators—Programmed instruction.
2. Arrhythmia—Programmed instruction.   3. Electrocardiography—Programmed
instruction.
  [DNLM: 1. Electrocardiography, Ambulatory—methods.   2. Cardiac
Pacing, Artificial.   3. Pacemaker, Artificial.   WG 140 H587sm 2004]   I.
Hesselson, Aaron B. Simplified interpretation of pacemaker ECGs.   II.
Title.
  RC684.E4H47 2004
  617.4'120645—dc22
                                                        2004017900

A catalogue record for this title is available from the British Library

Acquisitions: Steve Korn
Production: Julie Elliott and Alice Nelson
Set in 10/13pt Meridien by Graphicraft Limited, Hong Kong
Printed and bound in Chelsea, MI USA by Sheridan Books, Inc.

For further information on Blackwell Publishing, visit our website:
www.blackwellfutura.com

Notice: The indications and dosages of all drugs in this book have been recommended
in the medical literature and conform to the practices of the general community. The
medications described do not necessarily have specific approval by the Food and Drug
Administration for use in the diseases and dosages for which they are recommended.
The package insert for each drug should be consulted for use and dosage as approved
by the FDA. Because standards for usage change, it is advisable to keep abreast of
revised recommendations, particularly those concerning new drugs.

Contents

SECTION II | **CASE STUDIES**

SECTION III | **ANSWERS**

Preface

It was in the early 1980s that the implantable cardioverter defibrillator (ICD) was first introduced for the treatment of life-threatening ventricular arrhythmias. The first generation of ICD was large, by today's standards, the lead system had to be implanted via a thoracotomy approach, the generator was short-lived, and had limited anti-tachycardia therapies with no pacemaker capabilities. Since then the ICD system has become smaller, implantable via an endovascular route, longer living, and fully capable of tailored anti-tachycardia and bradycardia pacing functions. The initial indications for implantation have progressed from the survival of two cardiac arrests to that of significant VT, VF, and even certain types of medically refractory congestive heart failure. As a consequence of these expanded indications and the increasing number of implanted devices, the demand for individuals needed to understand their function is ever greater.

In contrast to a pacemaker system where an analysis of surface electro-cardiography is primarily relied upon, ICDs demand an understanding of the intracardiac electrogram (EGM) in order to evaluate their function. This is particularly relevant for the most recent generation of ICD that offers biventricular pacing capabilities and display some of the most complex troubleshooting issues. A firm knowledge of pacemaker function, EGM and electrocardiogram (ECG) analysis provides the foundation on which to begin this understanding. This text will proceed from there by demonstrating the basics of ICD. From this one should develop the essential skills needed to analyze these amazing cardiac devices.

Aaron B. Hesselson

Foreword

In the past two decades, the evolution of ICDs has revolutionized the treatment for primary and secondary prevention of sudden cardiac death. While early devices were nonprogrammable "shock" boxes using a single ventricular lead and required thoracic surgery for implantation, current devices are small (less than 30 cc), multiprogrammable, with either dual chamber or three chamber (biventricular) lead systems. These advances in technology have not only facilitated the ease of implantation of such systems, but have increased the indications and benefits of such devices. Thus, it is not surprising that there has been logorrhythmic growth in implantation if ICDs, such that nearly 150 000 new units will be expected to be implanted in 2004. The complexity of these devices has lead to an equally complex requirement for understanding their normal and abnormal function, both in diagnostic and therapeutic modalities.

Faced with an inordinate amount of information available on such devices, a simplified way to systematically approach an understanding of normal and abnormal function is needed. This is even more important as devices become implanted by non-electrophysiologists. Dr Hesselson has provided an immense service to implantors of devices and those people caring for patients with these devices. In this text, Dr Hesselson has put together a simple, yet thorough and lucid description of ICD technology and explanations of how they work both to sense and deliver therapies. Specific chapters are dedicated to understanding the hardware and the electronics of these systems. Additional chapters are related to the diagnostic components of the device (i.e. sensing and detection) and the therapies which can be delivered through such devices. Importantly, complications of the devices are discussed, as well as the influence of a variety of anti-arrhythmic agents on sensing, pacing, and defibrillation. The definitions of parameters used to understand the complexities are carefully explained in a very easy to understand style. Most important is the use of case studies to understand normal and abnormal function of these devices. Causes for inappropriate shocks or anti-tachycardia pacing, undersensing and oversensing are given by clear examples from real patients. The book is replete with well chosen interrogation strips as well as simplified diagrams to make obvious that which is truly complex.

Dr Hesselson is to be complimented for providing a simple to understand, extremely useful book on the basics of ICDs that will be of use to all cardiologists. His programmed teaching style is invaluable in helping all of us feel more comfortable in dealing with these complicated and increasingly widely employed devices.

Mark E. Josephson, MD
Herman C. Dana Professor of Medicine
Chief, Cardiovascular Division
Director, Harvard–Thorndike Electrophysiology
Institute and Arrhythmia Service

Acknowledgements

The following were instrumental influences, without whom this book would not have been possible: Robert Sorrentino, MD; Ruth Ann Greenfield, MD; Matthew Flemming, MD; Sue Pasko, RN; Susan Illikman, RN; the nursing staff of Eastlake Cardiovascular; the EP lab/OR staff of St John and Bon Secours Hospitals; and all of the industry personnel who shared in my enthusiasm for ICD troubleshooting.

SECTION I

ICD Basics

CHAPTER 1

What is an ICD?

What is an ICD?

An implantable cardioverter defibrillator (ICD) is an automatic electronic device primarily used to treat the arrhythmias ventricular tachycardia (VT) and ventricular fibrillation (VF). Quite often it is prescribed for patients whose ventricular heart muscle function has become severely compromised or those unfortunate to have been born with certain genetic defects that put them at risk for developing VT/VF. Like the permanent pacemaker, the current generation of ICD is typically inserted on the chest below the clavicle and may also provide pacemaker function to prevent the heart rhythm from becoming too slow and/or discoordinated. Unlike the pacemaker, an ICD's ultimate function is to prevent sudden cardiac death (SCD)* by delivering internal shock(s) to the heart when it determines that VT/VF has occurred. Rapid ventricular pacing may also be brought to bear for terminating slower varieties of VT.

1 An automatic implantable electronic device used to treat VT/VF is an

_____.

2 An ICD can prevent _____ by delivering a shock to terminate VT/VF.

---

* Death within 30 minutes of the onset of a cardiac event.

ICDs come in both ventricular and dual chamber varieties. Dual chamber ICDs also afford pacemaker function in the atrium, and may, depending on the brand, have the ability to treat paroxysms of atrial tachyarrhythmias with rapid pacing and cardioversion therapies.

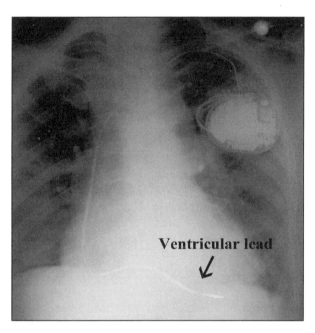

Ventricular lead

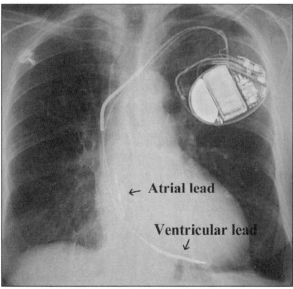

← Atrial lead

Ventricular lead

An ICD may also appear in what is called a "biventricular" type that has a left ventricular pacing lead in addition. Biventricular ICDs treat certain types of congestive heart failure through synchronous left and right ventricular pacing (see Chapter 9 for more details regarding biventricular pacing).

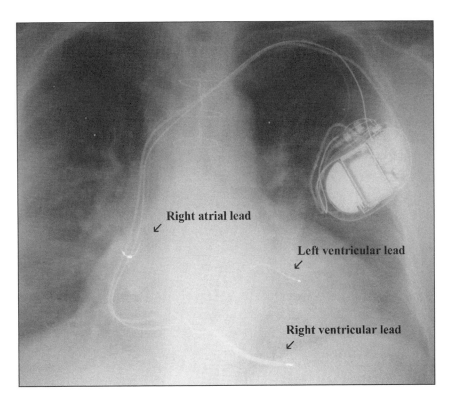

3 An ICD may appear in a _____, _____ chamber atrio-ventricular, and _____ -ventricular variety.

4 A biventricular ICD also treats _____ _____ _____.

CHAPTER 2

ICD System and Cardiac Anatomy

ICD System and Cardiac Anatomy

The lead(s) utilized for a contemporary ICD are implanted via the venous system beneath the clavicle in a similar manner to those of a pacemaker. Usually this occurs on the left side as this allows for the optimal path for defibrillating the heart. The tip of the ventricular defibrillator lead is typically placed in the apex of the right ventricle (RV). Whereas a ventricular pacemaker lead can potentially be placed anywhere in the RV that provides adequate pacing and sensing, the defibrillator lead optimally needs to be in the apex or not far away. This is because successful defibrillation is maximized by keeping as much of the left ventricular muscle within the shock path (vector) as possible. A ventricular lead placed more superiorly on the septal wall can cause ventricular muscle to appear outside the shocking vector and can lead to unsuccessful VT/VF termination. The atrial lead utilized for a dual chamber ICD is the same as that for a pacemaker and currently has no special limitations on positioning within the right atrium.

1 The tip of a defibrillator lead is most commonly placed in the RV_____.

2 The right atrial lead of a dual chamber ICD _____ have positioning limitations.

Should a left ventricular lead be desired to allow for biventricular pacing, it can be placed either within the left ventricular venous anatomy through the coronary sinus (CS):

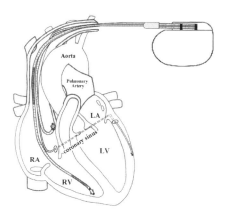

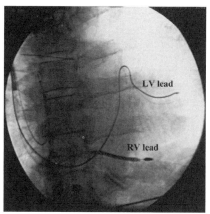

. . . or on the outside of the left ventricle (LV) during an open chest thoracotomy.

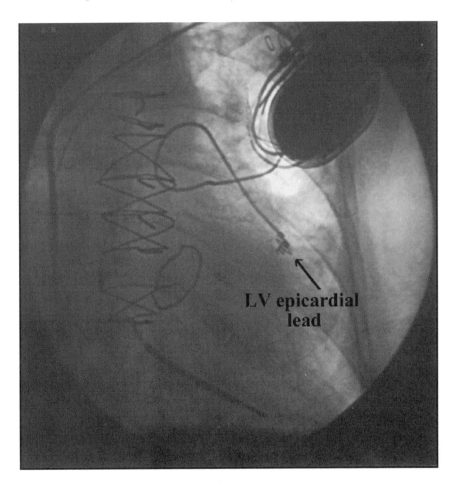

LV epicardial lead

Cardiac Venous Anatomy

The CS drains venous blood from the heart into the right atrium. Many branches from the LV flow into the CS, including those from the lateral and posterior LV. Currently, it is there that a left ventricular pacing lead is optimally placed. This may be best visualized under fluoroscopy from a left anterior oblique (LAO) perspective. Many patients who are candidates to receive a CS left ventricular lead, however, have had myocardial infarctions that may limit the ability to pace from these sites. Stimulation of the left phrenic nerve during ventricular pacing may occur, and can preclude placement there (the left phrenic nerve travels in close proximity to this cardiac region on its way to the left hemi-diaphragm).

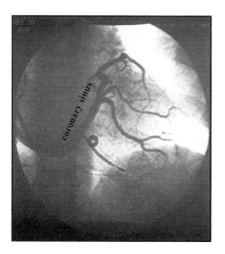 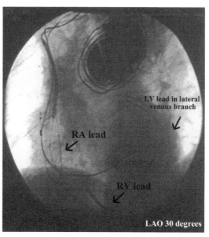

3 The CS drains blood into the _____ _____.

4 The _____ _____ travels in close proximity to the postero-lateral LV.

Also, the cardiac venous anatomy is extremely variable between individuals. Some may not have venous branches large enough to accept a pacemaker lead.

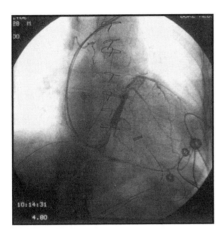 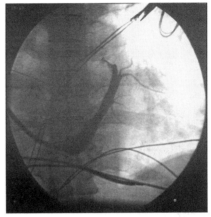

5 The anatomy of the cardiac venous system is extremely _____ between individuals.

CHAPTER 3

The Hardware

The Hardware

A complete ICD system consists of the ICD generator and lead(s).

The ICD Generator

The ICD generator has the necessary elements to coordinate all pacing, sensing, and defibrillation functions. These elements include the battery and electronic circuitry ("brains" and capacitor(s)).

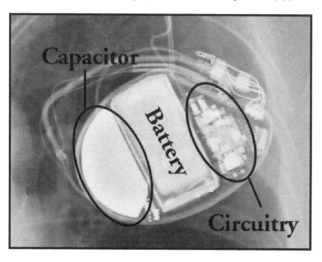

The Battery

Each ICD has a battery whose lifetime is dependent on how much pacing and defibrillating the device is called upon to perform. Typical longevities currently may fall between about 4–7 years.

As opposed to a pacemaker, whereby placement of a magnet causes it to pace asynchronously, this has no effect on pacing in the current generation of ICD. As such it has no "magnet rate" and needs to be interrogated at regular intervals in order to determine how much battery life there is. Placement of a magnet over an ICD, however, may actually turn off the delivery of anti-tachycardia therapies, and should only be performed by individuals experienced with this action.

The Circuitry

The ICD circuitry determines how and when both bradycardia pacing and anti-tachycardia therapies are delivered. The sophisticated circuitry facilitates a wide range of programming options, so that each device can be tailored to function in a manner most appropriate for each individual.

The ICD capacitor(s) is (are) a critical electrical element allowing for defibrillation. Capacitors perform this task by first storing energy ("charging") that can then be released in a path across the heart (defibrillation/cardioversion).

Advancements in battery and capacitor technology have permitted significant downsizing of the devices since their inception.

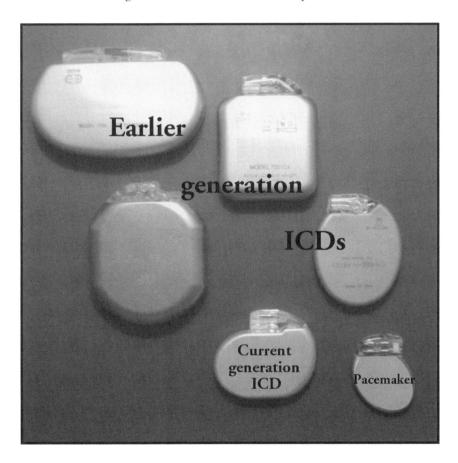

1 An ICD battery may last about _____ years.

2 A critical electronic element allowing for defibrillation is the _____.

The ICD Header and Can

The ICD generator communicates with the heart through a ventricular defibrillator ± atrial and LV electrode or "lead." The leads are connected to the ICD via a "header." The header provides holes for insertion of all aspects of the ventricular defibrillator lead and, if also needed, an atrial and LV lead in specific ICD models. As in the pacemaker, set screws in the header may be tightened to fix the leads in place or loosened to allow their removal.

The metal casing of the ICD generator is called the "can." The can is similar in composition to that of the pacemaker and will protect the ICD's electrical elements from fluids and many external electrical sources. However, cellular telephones and certain types of diagnostic and therapeutic medical equipment can interact with an ICD, or potentially cause harm to the device. The can may also function as an integral part of the defibrillation circuit (more on this in Chapter 4).

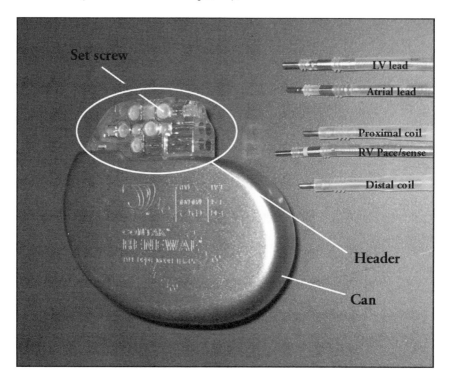

3 The ICD _____ allows for lead fixation.

4 The ICD _____ may play an active part in the defibrillation circuit.

Ventricular ICD Leads

A contemporary ventricular defibrillator lead consists of multiple internally separated metal wires that are externally encased in silicone rubber or polyurethane insulation. This allows the lead to function similarly to a standard pacemaker lead, i.e. transmission of electrical pacing/sensing signals between the heart and generator, but also structurally provides a separate pathway that participates in the delivery of shocks. This pathway includes what are commonly referred to as the lead "coil(s)." Shocks are delivered across the heart between the coil(s) and potentially the ICD can. Each element of the lead has its own pin that may connect to the ICD header.

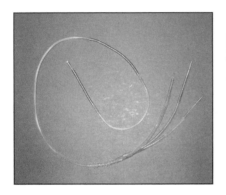
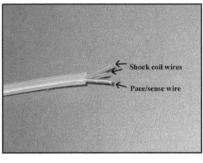

5 Each ventricular defibrillator lead has a pathway for _____/_____ and delivery of _____ energy.

6 The _____ may participate along with the _____(s) in shock delivery.

Ventricular ICD leads are commonly described by having the presence of one (single) or two (dual) coils. Both types have a coil distally, but a dual coil lead also has a proximal one along the length of the lead that preferably winds up in the superior vena cava (SVC) when this type of lead is desired. The type of lead chosen, dual or single coil, is dependent on the preference of the implanting physician and may be influenced by the patient's cardiac size and/or ejection fraction (more on the logic behind this choice in the Chapter 4 section on defibrillation pathways). Thus each ventricular defibrillator lead has a total of either two or three pins that connect to the ICD, one for pacing and sensing and one or two additional for defibrillating, depending on whether it is a single or dual coil lead.

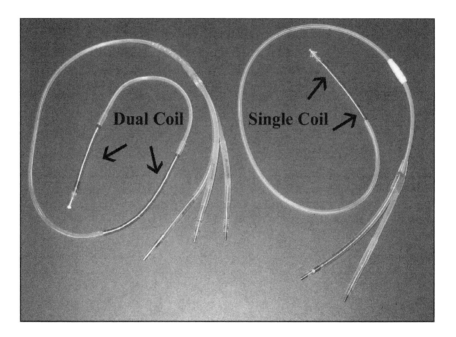

7 A defibrillator lead can be described by the presence of _____ or _____ coils.

8 A dual and single coil defibrillator lead have, respectively, _____ and _____ pins that connect to the ICD header.

As with pacemaker leads the ventricular ICD lead comes in both tined and screw-in varieties, but only in a bipolar configuration. There are, however, two types of bipolar configurations in common use, "integrated" and "true" bipolar.

An integrated bipolar configuration utilizes the lead tip and the distal coil for pacing and sensing purposes while a true bipolar configuration utilizes the tip and a ring electrode. As one might imagine, an integrated configuration provides for a larger window of sensing, and thus more opportunity for sensing non-cardiac potentials (i.e. diaphragmatic muscle potentials).

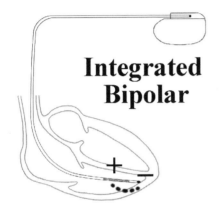

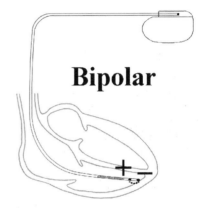

9 Two types of bipolar defibrillator leads, as described by their sensing configuration, are called _____ and _____ bipolar.

10 A true bipolar lead incorporates a _____ electrode.

As suggested earlier the proximal coil in a dual coil lead is optimally positioned in the SVC. Some patients' hearts may be so large that the proximal coil would not wind up there. One way to manage this situation, when a dual coil system is initially desired, is to rather utilize a single coil lead, but adding a lead called an "SVC coil" to the system. This is a separate lead that is connected to the proximal shocking coil port of the ICD and is independently positioned to float in the SVC. In other patients who develop an elevated defibrillation threshold (DFT) after initial implant of only a single coil lead, the SVC coil may also be subsequently added.

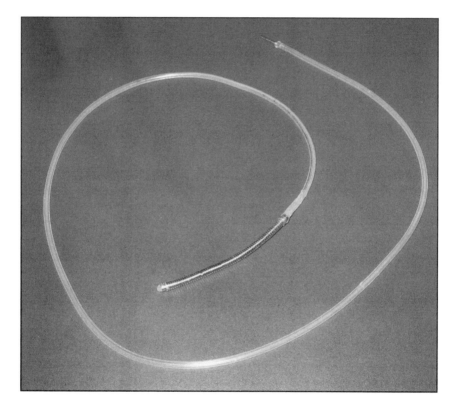

11 An _____ coil may be added to a single coil lead in an attempt to lower an elevated DFT.

Rarely, the ICD is unable to convert VF with an adequate safety margin despite an optimally positioned transvenous system. One way to improve this situation is to implant a "subcutaneous array or patch." Either provides another lead that can be connected to the ICD in place of the proximal shocking coil and can lower the energy level needed to convert VF. The patch or array is implanted underneath the skin and wrapped around the chest over where the LV lies. The pin is tunneled through the subcutaneous tissues to the pocket where the ICD sits.

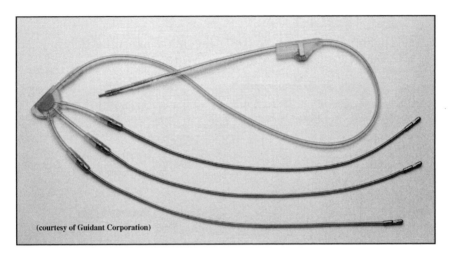

(courtesy of Guidant Corporation)

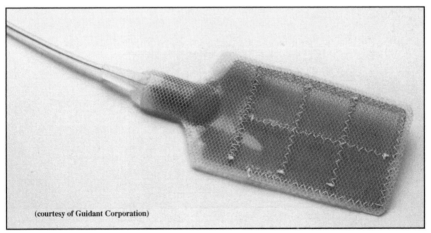

(courtesy of Guidant Corporation)

12 A subcutaneous _____ or _____ may be implanted as a means of lowering an elevated DFT.

13 When a subcutaneous device is used to improve DFT it takes the place of the _____ shocking coil in the ICD header.

A patient may rarely be encountered whose ICD system was originally implanted in the abdomen. The original ICD in such a system was
large. Part of this system could include "patch(es)" that were placed
directly over the surface of the heart from an open chest surgical procedure,

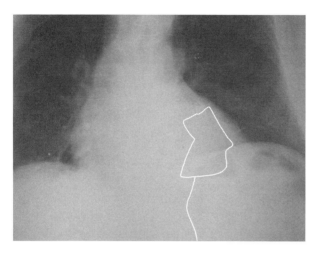

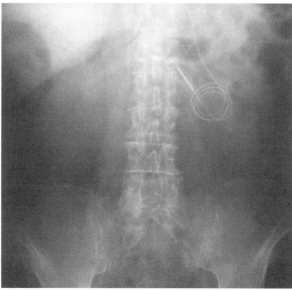

or a transvenous lead inserted at the shoulder.

These leads were then tunneled through the soft tissues to connect to the ICD in the abdomen.

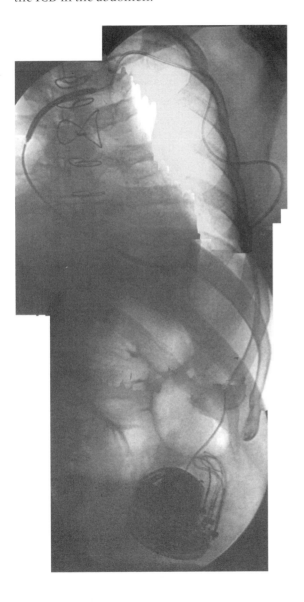

The ICD Programmer

Identical programmers are used for both pacemaker and ICD analysis. To facilitate this process, software particular to the ICD is loaded in the programmer in addition to the pacemaker software. Most programmers are smart and will automatically identify what type of device a patient has during interrogation, be it a pacemaker or ICD. It then downloads the appropriate software. This assumes, of course, that the programmer particular to the manufacturer of the ICD has been chosen. Once this is done telemetry is established between the ICD and programmer. All of the ICD settings are then available for review on the programmer screen or on paper by having the programmer print the information.

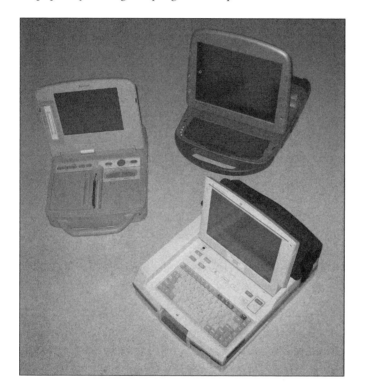

14 The _____ programmer may be used to interrogate both an ICD and pacemaker from one device manufacturer.

15 A programmer may _____ recognize what device it is interrogating, so long as the device and programmer are from the same manufacturer.

Programmer Telemetry

Once interrogation has been performed a vast amount of information is available for review. This includes how the ICD is set up to perform pacing functions and detect/deliver tachyarrhythmia therapies. Most devices allow a summary of the major functions to be printed in a short format.

					Apr 16, 2003 14:00:45	
ICD Model: Marquis DR 7274 — 9966 Software Version 3.0 — Serial Number: — Copyright — **Quick Look Report** — **Page 2**

Parameter Summary

Type Detection		Rx1	Rx2	Rx3	Rx4	Rx5	Rx6
VF	On	30 J	30 J	30 J	30 J	30 J	30 J
FVT	Off						
VT	Off						

SVT Criteria On: AF/Afl, Sinus Tach

Modes		Rates		A-V Intervals	
Mode	DDD	Lower	60 ppm	Paced AV	180 ms
Mode Switch	Off	Upper Track	120 ppm	Sensed AV	150 ms

Lead Parameters	Atrial	Ventricular
Amplitude	3 V	3 V
Pulse Width	0.4 ms	0.4 ms
Sensitivity	0.3 mV	0.3 mV

16 ICD interrogation allows one to determine how the device is set up to perform _____ and _____ functions.

As with pacemaker analysis an electrocardiogram (ECG) cable can be attached to the patient to provide ECG rhythm strips. They can aid in assessing the pacing and sensing functions of the ICD. "Marker channel" annotations are also available. They vary from those for pacemakers in that additional annotations are used to delineate ventricular events that occur within the various ICD tachycardia treatment zones (i.e. "VT" for VT zone or "VF" for VF zone for the below example). These tachycardia annotations differ between ICD manufacturers, but tend to convey similar information.

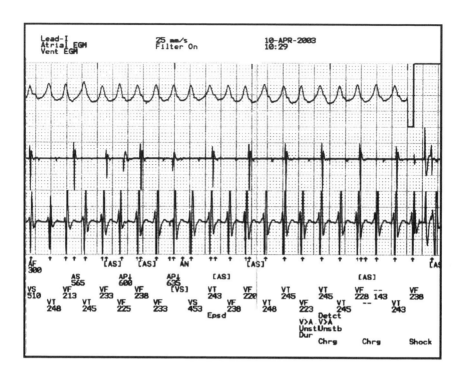

17 There are additional _____ on marker channels for heartbeats detected in an ICD tachycardia detection zone.

18 Tachycardia annotations may _____ between the manufacturers, but essentially convey the same information.

Electrograms (EGMs) are also available to display intracradiac signals of interest in real-time. Some ICDs allow one to choose from a number of EGM recording configurations. For example, an EGM can be measured between the bipolar electrodes in the ventricles and atria, between the shock coils (a so-called "shock" or "high voltage" EGM), and even between the atrial and ventricular lead components in dual chamber ICDs. For the purposes of this text the figure reference "VEGM" (ventricular EGM) assumes a recording is from the distal pair of ventricular lead electrodes.

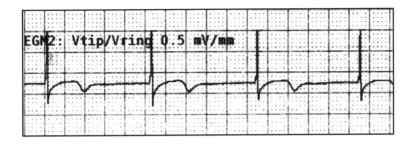

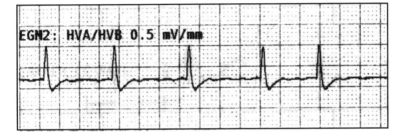

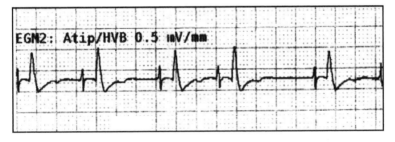

19 _____ may be recorded utilizing electrode sites in both the atria and ventricles.

The EGMs can be automatically recorded by the ICD when it determines that a significant tachycardia event has occurred. Event information may then be retrieved through device interrogation. This allows for a review of each event and an analysis of whether it was treated appropriately. Chapter 7 will go into greater detail regarding the EGM appearance of the tachycardias an ICD is likely to encounter.

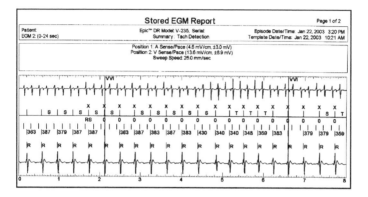

The ICD also keeps a running tally of the number of events it has recorded. This includes the number of times it has been required to render treatment as well as the number of events that it has detected.

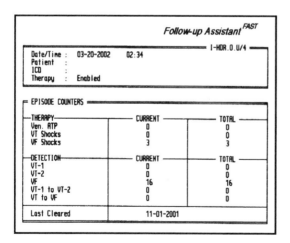

20 A tachycardia _____ is often automatically recorded by an ICD and available for review.

21 An event report is available for review by _____ an ICD.

Non-Invasive Programmed Stimulation/Electrophysiologic Study

Once an ICD has been implanted it becomes necessary to evaluate its ability to successfully convert VF. In order to do so, VF needs to be induced. This is easily accomplished as each manufacturer's programmer has some form of non-invasive programmed stimulation (NIPS) or electrophysiologic study (EPS) feature that allows the programmer to direct stimulation commands to the heart through the ICD. Such options as a low energy "shock-on-T wave" or high frequency ventricular burst pacing can induce VF. One only needs to select the desired option on the programmer screen. A command is then transmitted to the ICD to perform. The ICD is allowed to deliver its treatment once it has detected the arrhythmia.

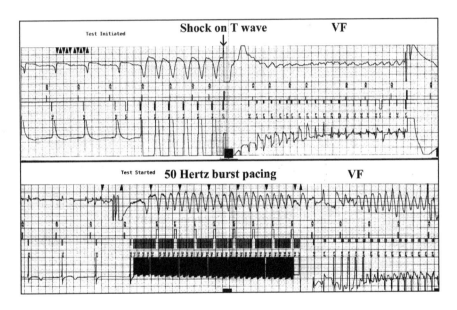

22 VF may be _____ by an ICD through commands directed from the programmer.

23 A _____ -on- _____ wave feature is one means of VF induction.

Another form of programmed stimulation allows ventricular extra-stimuli to be delivered through the ICD system in the same protocol as one would do with a ventricular catheter inserted from the groin and connected to an external stimulator. Some physicians may use this feature as a means of attempting arrhythmia induction and evaluating the efficacy of anti-tachycardia overdrive pacing for VT. This practice, however, is becoming less commonplace. All of the above non-invasive stimulation maneuvers are performed under appropriate patient sedation and with external defibrillator back-up.

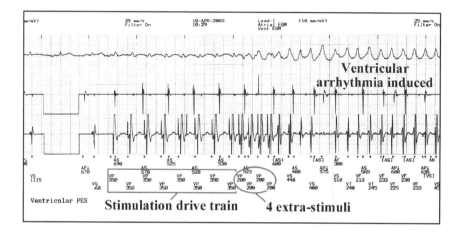

24 Ventricular _____ -stimuli may delivered from an ICD by commands from the programmer.

25 Non-invasive stimulation maneuvers are always performed with adequate patient _____ and an external back-up _____.

CHAPTER 4

ICD Electronics

ICD Electronics

The ICD can be thought of as having two major electrical circuits, one being for pacing/sensing and the other for cardioversion/defibrillation.* The pacing/sensing circuit functions in a similar manner as that in a pacemaker, and is subject to the identical principals relating voltage, current, and resistance/impedance.

In review, the ventricular ICD lead and heart provide an impedance (Z) to the flow of current (I) when connected to a voltage (V) source (the ICD generator). As current flows the heart can then be stimulated (paced).

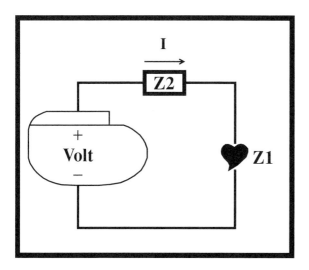

1 An ICD can be thought of as having two major electrical circuits, one for _____/_____ and the other for _____/_____.

2 The same principals relating voltage, current, and resistance/impedance may be applied to a pacemaker and _____.

---

* For simplification, this will subsequently be referred to as the defibrillation circuit throughout this chapter.

The heart also acts as a voltage source that can cause current to flow with each beat and register a signal in the ICD's sensing circuitry. This information can then be used to inhibit pacing, and also provide input to the defibrillator circuit.

The initial voltage of the contemporary ICD battery is typically between about 3–6 volts (V). Impedance values for a ventricular defibrillator pacing lead system tend to be in the range of about 200–1000 ohms (Ω). Just like a pacemaker circuit, however, changes in impedance during ventricular pacing over time may indicate a structural malfunction in the pacing/sensing portion of the defibrillator lead (i.e. a higher impedance may indicate a fracture and a lower impedance an insulation defect).

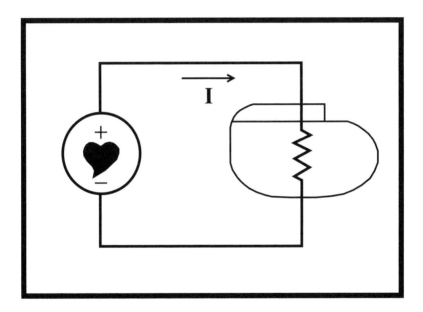

3 Ventricular sensing in an ICD is used to _____ pacing and provides _____ to the defibrillation circuit.

4 A pacing impedance level of about _____ to _____ohms is typical for a ventricular defibrillator lead.

Defibrillator Circuit

A very simplified version of an ICD defibrillator circuit can be described as having a voltage source (ICD battery), resistance/impedance source (ICD shocking coil(s), ICD resistors, and heart), and charge reservoir (capacitor(s)*). When connected to a voltage source, a capacitor stores a charge and develops its own voltage potential as current flows. This is a process called "charging." Over a very short period of time (seconds) the ICD capacitor may develop a potential of 800+ V. This amount of voltage is necessary to generate the energy levels required for defibrillation.

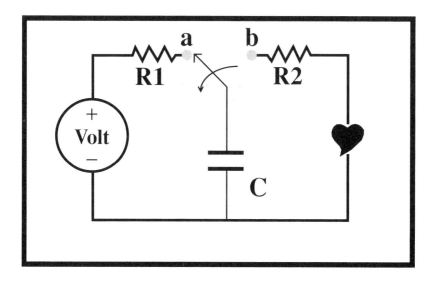

5 A capacitor develops a _____ potential as it stores _____.

6 The time period that a capacitor charges is measured in _____.

---

* A specialized electrical element that stores charge. Some ICDs have two as opposed to one capacitor.

The capacitor voltage for this simplified circuit may then be described by the exponential equation:

V capacitor $= (V$ ICD battery$)\, e^{-t/RC}$

(t = time, R = resistance, C = capacitance; measured in microfarads (μF); 10^{-6} Farads)

The energy stored in the capacitor for a given level of charged voltage is:

Energy $= {}^{1}/_{2}\, CV^{2}$

For example, an ICD with an effective capacitance of 125 μF may charge to 800 V in about 6–10 seconds. The energy stored in the capacitor equals $^{1}/_{2}$ **(125 × 10^{-6}) × (800)^{2}** or **40 Joules (J)**. What is important about these equations is that it takes time for the ICD battery to charge the capacitor (i.e. the higher the voltage required, and thus the higher the energy, then the longer the charge time), and the value of capacitance times resistance in the charging circuit affects the manner in which charging occurs.

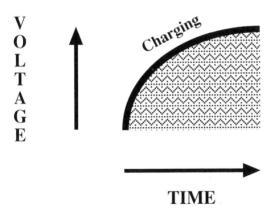

**V
O
L
T
A
G
E**

Charging

TIME

7 Charging a capacitor takes _____.

8 The energy stored in a capacitor equals $^{1}/_{2}$ the product of capacitance and the square of the _____.

Once the desired amount of energy is stored in the capacitor the contents may be "discharged" with the heart being in the path of the ICD shock. The discharge of the capacitor also follows an exponential path. For practical purposes this is how defibrillation is accomplished by the ICD (the circuitry is much more complex in actuality, but the principles described are very applicable). The impedance in this portion of the circuit is low (about 25–100 Ω) which allows for a rapid delivery of the capacitor's contents. Should the "shock impedance"* change over time this may indicate a problem with the ventricular defibrillator lead (i.e. increased impedance suggests shock coil fracture vs. decreased impedance suggests an insulation defect).

ICD capacitors periodically undergo automatic charging without delivery of energy to the patient. This is a process called capacitor "auto-reformation." It helps maintain the efficiency of capacitor function.

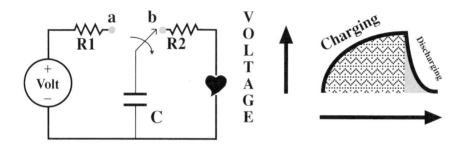

9 Typical shock impedances are between _____ and _____ohms.

10 An increased shock impedance over time may indicate a _____ in the shock coil circuit.

---

* Not to be confused with the pacing lead impedance. Each impedance value, shock and lead, may independently change should a lead problem effect the pacing vs. the shocking circuit, and vice versa.

Defibrillation Waveforms

The first ICDs delivered their shocks in what may be described as a "monophasic" configuration. All of the energy was delivered in one polarity, an initial or reversed polarity.

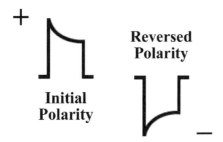

Subsequent generations of ICDs have taken advantage of the greater efficacy of a "biphasic" shock configuration for converting ventricular tachyarrhythmias. Here each shock is split into two portions of opposite polarities minimally separated in time.

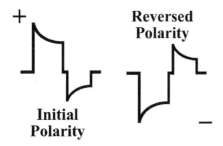

One may note that the above shock waveforms do not appear the same as the capacitor waveform shown before. In actuality, there is electrical manipulation of the shock waveform to more resemble those above.

11 A monophasic shock has _____ component.

12 A _____ shock waveform has two portions of opposite polarity minimally separated in time.

Defibrillation Shock Polarity and Configuration

The polarity in which an ICD shock is delivered is programmable in most conventional devices (initial or reversed polarity). Selecting a shock polarity comes into play when testing shock efficacy. One polarity may be successful when the other is not. Thus, when successful VF defibrillation is not accomplished to an adequate safety margin with one shock polarity a reversal of polarity is usually attempted first. This simple maneuver may yield an appropriate shock safety margin and negate the need to implant further hardware. Also, successful defibrillation is more likely to occur when the amount of left ventricular myocardium in the shock pathway is maximized. To this end some pathways and lead configurations may work better than others.

In conventional ICD systems the can may participate in the shocking circuit (called a "hot can" or "active can"). For a single coil lead system each ICD shock occurs between the right ventricular coil and the can. This configuration may work well in many instances, but in patients with larger and more poorly functioning hearts a physician may choose not to use a single coil lead as it may not provide an adequate shocking vector or "defibrillation threshold."

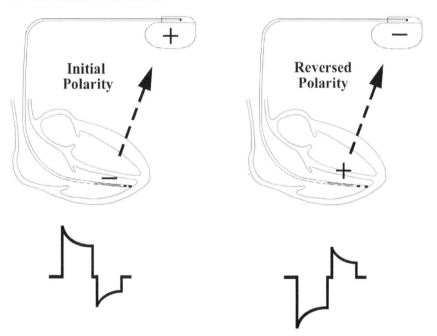

13 When the amount of left ventricular myocardium in a shock pathway is _____ successful rhythm conversion is more likely.

14 A "can" that participates in a shock is called a _____ _____ or _____ _____.

Defibrillation Threshold

The defibrillation threshold (DFT) is the amount of energy required to consistently convert VF. The term DFT is actually a misnomer as there is not a true threshold at which defibrillation success will always occur. Whether or not VF is converted is actually a function of dose–response, i.e. the higher the energy level then the more likely VF will be converted. Because of this, multiple initiations of VF are commonly performed (two times or more) during initial ICD implantation. If successful conversion at energy levels at least 10 J less than the maximum energy output of the ICD are consistently observed this helps to ensure that the likelihood of future successful conversion is maximized when a 10 J "safety margin" is programmed.

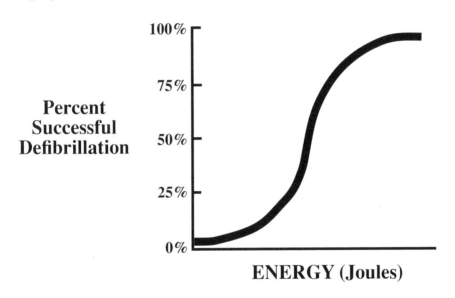

15 Successful defibrillation is a function of _____–_____.

16 A commonly accepted safety margin for defibrillation is _____.

Should a single coil lead configuration not yield an adequate DFT even after polarity reversal, or it is felt by the physician that the proximal coil of a dual coil lead would not be optimally placed in the SVC, a separate SVC coil can be added to the system. Here both coils and the ICD can may participate in the shock pathway and lower the DFT.

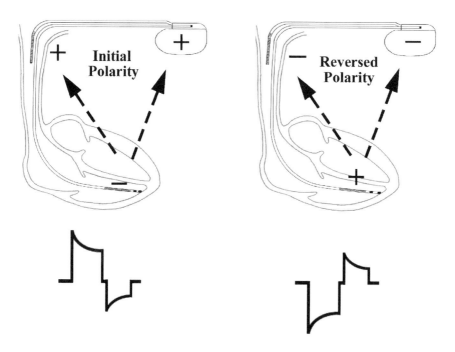

17 An _____ coil may be added to a single coil ICD lead as an attempt to lower the DFT.

With a dual coil lead similar defibrillation shock pathways can be duplicated as with a single coil lead plus SVC coil. This assumes, as mentioned before, that the proximal coil is in the SVC.

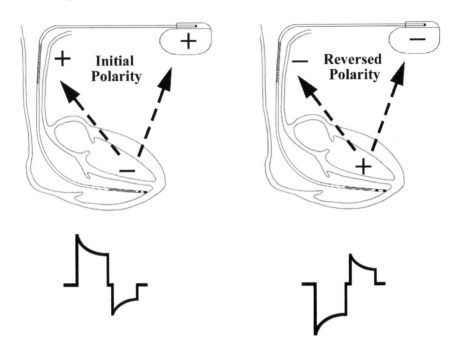

18 A dual coil lead may yield a _____ DFT than a single coil lead.

In some ICD models the can may be programmed out of the shock pathway, if desired.

Can inactivated

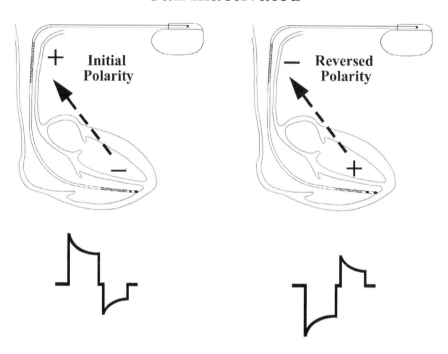

19 The _____ may be programmed out of a shock pathway in some ICD models.

Even with an appropriately positioned dual coil system and attempts using both shock polarities the DFT may rarely remain unacceptably high. In this instance the implanting physician has the option of taking the proximal coil out of the defibrillation circuit and adding a subcutaneous array or patch as a means of improving the DFT.

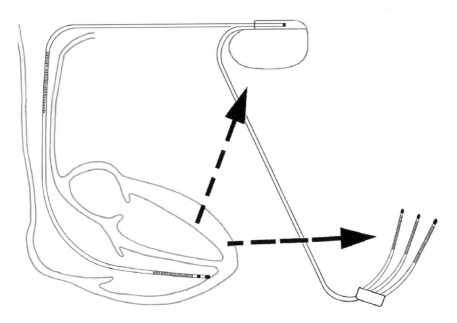

The need for a subcutaneous device is not very common, however. This may be due in part to the ability to typically achieve adequate DFTs with endovascular leads, and the availability of "high energy" ICDs that may offer up to 42 J of stored energy.

20 A subcutaneous _____ or _____ may lower an unacceptably high DFT.

21 "_____ energy" ICDs may obviate the addition of a subcutaneous device due to an elevated DFT.

CHAPTER 5

Sensing

Sensing in an ICD is quite dissimilar to that in a pacemaker. Why? Recall that the R wave signals of a typical pacemaker system may fall between about 5–25 millivolt (mV). In contrast, an ICD needs to be able to detect VF wavelets that may be of very small amplitude, on the order of tenths of a millivolt. Simply setting a fixed sensitivity level at such a low level in an ICD without any other adjustments would likely cause T wave over-sensing in any baseline rhythm. A ventricular refractory period would not solve this issue as the ICD needs to be alert during this time period for any tachycardia events.

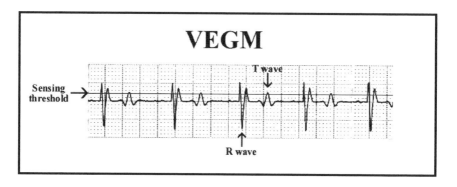

As such appropriate sensing in an ICD system, and thus appropriate detection of ventricular tachyarrhythmias, rests on the ability to ignore signals such as T waves, while being able to recognize VF wavelets of a very small amplitude. Electronic filtering of lower frequency signals (i.e. T waves) is one such measure. How else is this accomplished?

1 VF wavelets are on the order of _____ of a millivolt in amplitude.

2 Appropriate ventricular sensing in an ICD relies upon the ability to ignore _____ waves.

An "auto-adjusting sensitivity" threshold that decreases throughout each cardiac cycle, while maintaining a fixed signal gain is one such strategy (Medtronic, current generation St Jude, Biotronik). Essentially with this method, the sensitivity threshold decreases over time following each sensed/paced event until either the maximum sensitivity (lowest threshold) is reached or the next sensed/paced event occurs. The sensitivity level then returns to a higher point that may be determined by the amplitude of the sensed R wave or a whether a paced event has occurred. The Medtronic sensitivity threshold follows an exponential-like decay path while the St Jude method follows a linear decline, and the Biotronik method a step-wise decline. Other methods that essentially fix the sensing threshold but amplify signal gain include (i) an "automatic gain control" scheme that steadily increases the signal gain after each paced/sensed event with each cardiac cycle (Guidant), and (ii) a beat-to-beat gain adjustment method that fixes signal gain for each cardiac cycle, but allows the gain to be altered after each ventricular complex based upon the amplitude of the prior signal (older St Jude models). As ICD technology progresses and improves, so too may these methodologies for ventricular sensing.

Auto-Adjusting Sensitivity

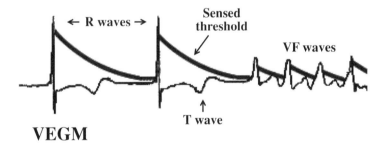

Automatic Gain Control

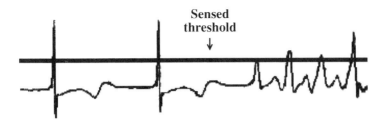

Sensing in the atria for dual chamber ICD models utilizes the same methodology as that in the ventricles in the current generation of devices.

3 Methods of sensing in an ICD include _____-_____ and automatic _____ control.

4 Contemporary ICD atrial sensing utilizes the _____ methodology as ventricular sensing.

CHAPTER 6

Detection

In order for an ICD to deliver a therapy it has to first be able to detect when a significant tachycardia is happening. The foundation on which this process occurs is a beat-by-beat analysis of heart rate. Multiple other factors or "discriminators" may be added to this analysis in order to make a proper determination of whether a tachycardia is of ventricular or supra-ventricular origin. This is particularly relevant for "slower" tachycardias. "Faster" rhythms are more likely to cause hemodynamic intolerance and are primarily detected by their rate only. Thus differences in heart rate allow multiple levels or "zones" of detection to be established in an ICD. In fact an ICD may be programmed with as many as three zones of detection, a single "VF zone" and two "VT zones." The zones are defined by pro-grammable rate cutoffs that are determined by the implanting physician. All ICDs have at least a VF zone. Whether or not a VT zone is programmed may be guided by the presence of a clinical VT in the patient. Why even have multiple zones of detection? This allows for different levels of therapy based on the zone of tachycardia detection.

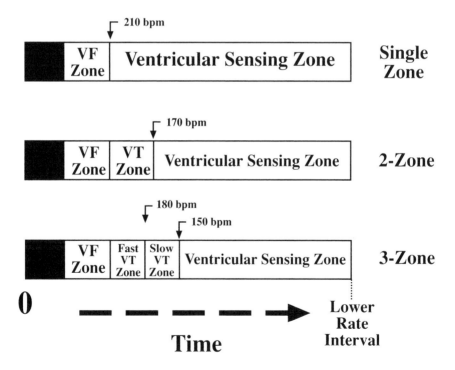

The methods for detection are not uniform amongst the ICD manufacturer's devices. Each has a specific methodology for establishing tachycardia detection and applying enhancements allowing for supraventricular tachycardia (SVT)/VT discrimination. The detection principles that follow are applicable to most ICDs and should provide a basis for understanding this process. One may refer to the physician's manual for detection nuances specific to each ICD manufacturer and model.

1 Tachycardia detection in an ICD is founded on a beat-by-beat analysis of _____ _____.

2 A contemporary ICD may have as few as _____, and as many as _____ zones of tachycardia detection for ventricular tachyarrhythmias.

3 Multiple tachycardia detection zones in an ICD allows for different levels of _____.

4 Tachycardia detection methods _____ between the various manufacturer's devices.

Heartbeat Classification

Each sensed ventricular heartbeat undergoes a classification determined by its relationship in time to the previous sensed/paced ventricular beat, and the number of zones of detection that have been programmed. "Time zero" below marks the point of initial pacing or sensing. An absolute refractory period (■) serves to prevent this beat from being sensed should it be a ventricular paced complex, or from being sensed a second time should the complex be a particularly wide native beat.

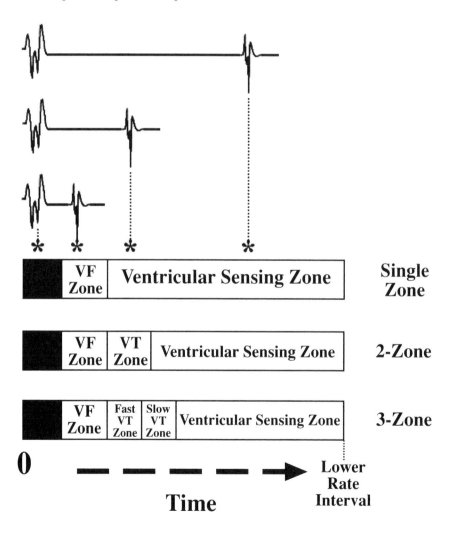

Thus as time passes a sensed heartbeat may fall into (i) a VF zone and be counted as a "VF" event, (ii) a VT zone, if present, and be counted as a "VT" event, or (iii) a ventricular sensing zone and be counted as a "VS" event.* Once a beat is classified this process is repeated for each subsequent sensed ventricular heartbeat. Classification in a St Jude ICD also takes into account an average of the time interval of the three prior heartbeats in order to assign a ventricular heartbeat into a VF, VT, or VS zone. If enough beats are classified over time in a VF and/or VT zone, then the initial criterion for tachycardia detection may be satisfied. What constitutes "enough beats" is determined by the manner that the ICD counts and how the ICD has been programmed.

5 Each ventricular heartbeat sensed by an ICD is _____ by which zone it falls into.

6 Where a heartbeat falls may depend on how many ICD _____ of detection have been programmed.

7 The ICD manufacturers may have _____ methods for classifying heartbeats.

8 _____ rhythm that is fast enough to fall into an ICD tachycardia detection zone has the potential to be _____.

---

* Just because a beat occurs in a VF or VT zone does not necessarily mean it is actually a beat of VF or VT. **ANY** rhythm whose rate is sufficient to cause its ventricular beats to fall into a tachycardia zone has the potential to be detected.

Methods of Counting

1 "Consecutive Interval Counting"

As its name implies, a consecutive interval counting scheme requires that a certain number of ventricular beats occur consecutively and are classified to a tachycardia zone in order to satisfy detection criterion. This number is programmable. For example if the number of beats needed to detect is 10, then 10 **consecutive** tachycardia beats are required to satisfy detection. Each interspersed non-tachycardia beat causes counting to be reset to zero. It is common to find this method of counting in VT detection zones. Exceptions include Guidant ICD models that utilize an "X of Y" counting method in their VT zones of detection, and Medtronic models where the physician has the choice of a consecutive interval or an "X of Y" counting scheme in the "Fast" VT zone.

9 A _____ interval counting method may commonly be used in a _____ detection zone.

10 A physician may _____ the number of intervals needed to detect in a tachycardia zone.

11 Counting in a consecutive interval scheme is reset to _____ when a non-tachycardia beat occurs.

2 "X of Y" Counting

This method of counting utilizes a continuous rolling window of detection that is updated with each new ventricular heartbeat. Detection is initially satisfied when X number out of the total number of beats in the window Y are classified to a tachycardia zone. For example, if an ICD detection window has a rolling detection window of 10 beats, it might require eight of those beats to be classified as VF in order to initially satisfy detection criterion. Why use this method of counting as opposed to a consecutive interval counting method? In particular VF may at times become extremely small in amplitude on the VEGM. As such there may be small gaps during the rhythm when the ICD does not classify a VF event. So as not to delay detection and treatment the X of Y method compensates for this possibility.

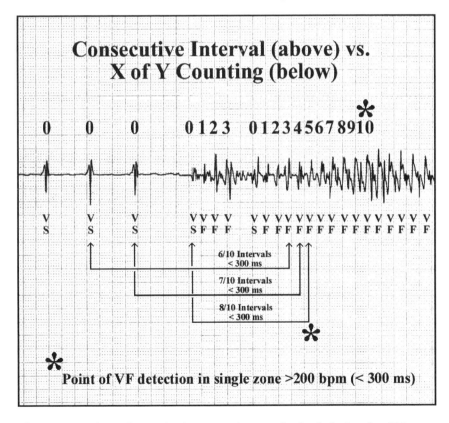

Thus, an X of Y scheme is the counting method of choice for VF zone detection. Also, VT can have some variation in its cycle length. An X of Y counting method may compensate for potential transient drops below the rate cutoff and prevent delayed detection and delivery of therapy.

SVT/VT Discriminators or Detection Enhancements

If heart rate was the only criterion for tachycardia detection then ICD therapy might be inappropriately delivered with each occurrence of an SVT with a rapid ventricular response. As such, heart rate is not the only factor that detection in VT zones may be reliant upon. Recognition of rapid SVTs may be facilitated with what are referred to as discriminators or detection enhancements. When programmed on they will cause therapy to be withheld, despite a sufficient rate for detection, should an SVT be indicated. Common enhancements include "sudden onset," "stability," electrogram width, and R wave morphology comparison. These will be described in detail in Chapter 7. Also, the addition of atrial rate information in dual chamber ICDs allows the relationship of atria and ventricle to be compared, further enhancing rhythm discrimination. ICD manufacturers have capitalized on these relationships and enhancements to devise complex algorithms for SVT/VT discrimination (i.e. "PR Logic" (Medtronic), "SMART Detection" (Biotronik)). Despite such strategies, an SVT may rarely cause an ICD to deliver therapy for what it thinks is a significant ventricular tachyarrhythmia. This might also occur when such parameters as a "sustained duration timer" (Guidant), "sustained VT timer" (Biotronik), or "high rate timeout" (Medtronic) feature are programmed. These features will override any detection enhancement from withholding therapy should a tachycardia be of a prolonged nature.

Because faster rhythms have a greater likelihood of causing hemodynamic intolerance detection enhancements are not usually applied in a VF detection zone where a rapid delivery of therapy is essential.

12 An _____ counting method is commonly found in a VF detection zone.

13 _____ or detection _____ may help differentiate VT from an SVT.

Rhythm Confirmation

An ICD may confirm that a tachycardia is sustained and has not spontaneously terminated after detection has occurred. If the ICD determines that spontaneous termination has occurred, then it will not deliver therapy. If the capacitor(s) has (have) charged the ICD may hold the energy in them until it is determined that the tachycardia has not quickly restarted. This facilitates a rapid delivery of a shock in case the tachycardia swiftly restarts.

Confirmation may occur immediately after capacitor charging has completed or during and immediately after capacitor charging depending on the ICD model. The exact criteria used to establish spontaneous arrhythmia termination differs between ICD models. Should an ICD be programmed for a "committed" shock, however, the confirmation process does not occur and the shock is delivered at the completion of capacitor charging even if the tachycardia has terminated. A committed shock may also occur for a tachycardia that has spontaneously terminated during confirmation but has quickly recurred and been detected.

Redetection

Once a therapy has been delivered the ICD makes a determination of whether the tachycardia episode has been successfully terminated. Criterion for redetection of an unsuccessfully terminated tachycardia may be less rigorous than that for initial detection. Following a shock redetection typically begins after an extended refractory period (on the order of 500–1000 ms). This period serves to prevent the shock energy itself from being detected as a ventricular event.

Bradycardia Pacing During Tachycardia Detection

The pacing mode may temporarily switch to a VVI or DDI back-up mode when a tachycardia has been detected.

14 Spontaneous termination of a detected tachycardia may cause an ICD to _____ the delivery of therapy.

15 _____ of the rhythm status may take place after or both during and after capacitor charging, depending on the ICD model.

16 The rhythm confirmation process is bypassed when shocks are _____.

17 _____ rigorous detection criterion may be applied for tachycardias that have not been successfully terminated following the delivery of a therapy.

18 An automatic pacing mode _____ may occur when a tachycardia has been detected.

CHAPTER 7

The Tachycardias

In order to understand how an ICD functions it is helpful to know how the typical tachycardias encountered by it may appear to its sensing circuitry. Only by doing so can one appreciate the difficulty the ICD has in differentiating SVT from VT. In fact both SVT and VT may look remarkably similar, especially to a single chamber ICD. Thus, an ICD may occasionally deliver therapy for an SVT because it can't differentiate SVT from VT. The challenge for the person performing the EGM interpretation, in order to make a proper assessment of function, is often to determine what the arrhythmia recorded by the ICD during an event was. Most often only intracardiac EGMs are available. Thus, in order to perform proper assessments one needs to make the transition from analyzing surface ECGs to intracradiac EGMs. What follows are surface lead rhythm strips of the more commonly encountered tachycardias with the actual atrial and/or ventricular intracradiac signal(s) from the distal recording bipoles as one might expect them to appear to both a dual and single chamber ICD. Also, the common SVT/VT discriminators are also described as they might relate to each rhythm. As mentioned earlier, there are discriminator/algorithm functions particular to an ICD manufacturer. These are not emphasized here. One is encouraged to review such features as needed in the appropriate ICD physician's manual.

Sinus Tachycardia

The normal rate response to exertion and stress is for the sinus heart rate to increase. When the rate is > 100 b.p.m. this is "sinus tachycardia," by definition. The increase in heart rate is typically not sudden, but rather usually displays a progressive acceleration up to a level dictated by the workload or stress. This rate can become quite rapid, even to the point of entering the tachycardia detection zone of the ICD. As regards the appearance to the ICD and the person interpreting, the VEGM R wave morphology most often remains the same during tachycardia as that during the baseline rhythm. An exception for sinus tachycardia, and any other SVT for that matter, is during what is called "rate related Bundle Branch Aberrancy (BBA)" (more on this a bit later).

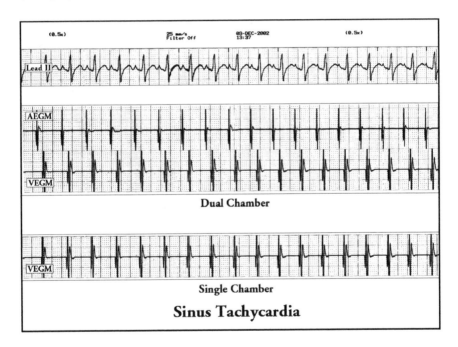

Dual Chamber

Single Chamber

Sinus Tachycardia

1 The onset of sinus tachycardia is typically not _____.

2 The VEGM R wave morphology during sinus tachycardia and normal sinus rhythm is typically the _____.

So how can the ICD differentiate sinus tachycardia from VT? Most ICDs can be programmed in their VT zones with a discriminator commonly referred to as "sudden onset." This can be used to help limit delivery of therapy for sinus tachycardia. Sudden onset tries to take advantage of the fact that sinus tachycardia, as opposed to VT, typically does not initiate in a sudden fashion. Other SVTs, however, can typically initiate in a sudden manner. In any case, an ICD may rarely deliver therapy for sinus tachycardia simply by the fact that a sustained rate criteria has been met should such a function be programmed on (it is actually quite common for both a sudden onset and sustained duration feature to be programmed on simultaneously).

Some ICDs may utilize comparisons of the baseline rhythm R wave morphology or width to that during tachycardia as a means of limiting inappropriate shocks for an SVT. For a morphology comparison each sensed beat undergoes an analysis from which the ICD assigns a percent match to that of a baseline template developed from the patient's normal rhythm. An SVT is considered likely when the R wave from the baseline template and those during tachycardia are matched to a great enough percentage.

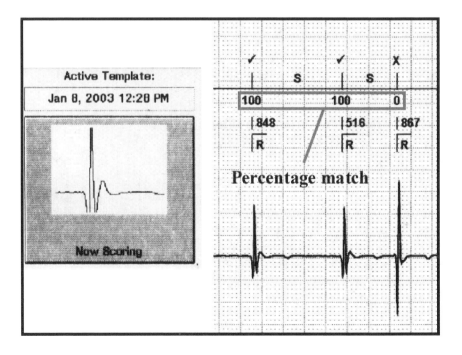

A comparison of R wave width may suggest an SVT when the tachycardia and baseline measurements are similar. Conversely a significant increase in width may suggest VT. The baseline width is developed from a sampling of many R waves during the patient's normal rhythm. The sampling is commonly from R waves as recorded by the shocking coils.

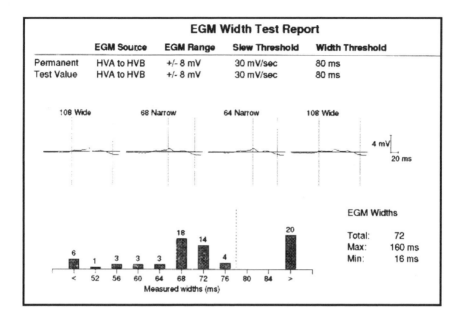

As such, these discriminators can be considered for helping to differentiate sinus tachycardia (or any other SVT for that matter) from VT. This is particularly relevant in single chamber ICDs (dual chamber ICDs may not have such features available). However, the phenomenon of BBA during SVT can "fool" such discriminators.

3 _____, _____, and _____ onset discriminators can help differentiate sinus tachycardia from VT.

Bundle Branch Aberrancy

As an SVT causes signal input below the atrio-ventricular (AV) node at progressively more rapid rates one of the bundle branches may cease conducting temporarily due to its refractory period being reached. What can happen then is the R wave morphology recorded by the ventricular defibrillator lead may change due to the alteration in ventricular activation.

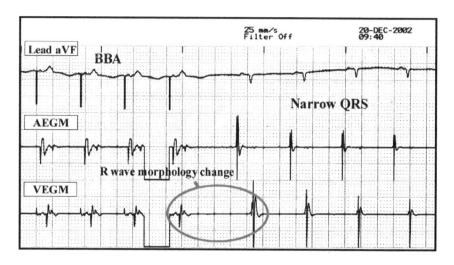

4 When its _____ period is reached a bundle branch may stop conducting.

5 _____ _____ morphology may change due to BBA.

Atrial Tachycardia

Atrial tachycardia (AT) is a rapid ectopic rhythm originating in one of the atria. The onset tends to be sudden. Its rate is usually found between about 130–240 b.p.m., and the rhythm may conduct in a 1 : 1 fashion to the ventricles. Thus, the rapidly conducted varieties may likely enter the detection zone(s) of the ICD. The atrial electrogram (AEGM) P wave morphology for a dual chamber ICD may show a noticeable change with the onset tachycardia, while the VEGM should remain the same absent BBA.

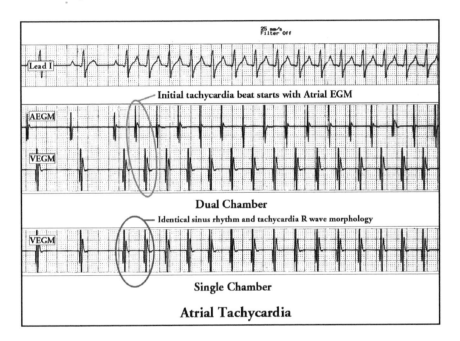

6 The onset of atrial tachycardia may be _____ and conduct in a _____ fashion to the ventricles.

When AT, and other tachycardias for that matter, is recorded as an event by the ICD the initiation may not be seen because the tachycardia rate may not initially fall in the detection zone. This is because it is not uncommon for some arrhythmias to "warm up" with slower rates followed by a faster one after some seconds have passed. If the arrhythmia onset is recorded then the EGM interpreter should pay notice that AT is typically initiated with an early atrial beat.

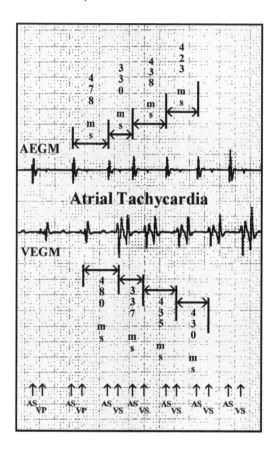

It may be difficult to differentiate a slower AT from VT with retrogradely conducted P waves. Changes in the atrial cycle length that precede and predict the subsequent change in ventricular cycle length favor AT (i.e. the atria "lead" the ventricles). Cycle length changes during tachycardia, however, may not always be obvious.

7 An arrhythmia may _____ _____ before accelerating to a faster rate.

8 Atrial cycle length changes during tachycardia that _____ and _____ ventricular cycle length changes favors AT over VT as the diagnosis.

A sudden onset function will not likely be of much use for the ICD to discriminate AT from VT since both can initiate in this fashion. A ventricular morphology or width discriminator may help, again in the absence of BBA. Not all ATs conduct each beat to the ventricles, so this information (# P waves > # R waves) in a dual chamber ICD event recording may allow the interpreter to help rule in the diagnosis of SVT. It should be noted that dual tachycardias, i.e. SVT and VT, can coexist in which the number of registered P waves is still greater then the number of registered R waves.

9 An atrial tachycardia may not conduct each _____ to the ventricles.

10 _____ tachycardias, i.e. SVT and VT, can coexist.

Typical AV Node Reentrant Tachycardia

AV node reentrant tachycardia (AVNRT) is one of the more common SVTs, and can occasionally be found in patients who have an ICD. The ability to develop this rhythm is dependent on there being two functional AV node pathways with different conduction properties. The "typical," and most common, form of AVNRT occurs when conduction proceeds from atria to ventricles down only a "slow" AV node pathway and returns back to the atria via a "fast" pathway during tachycardia (think of this as an electric circuit sort of like a dog chasing its tail about the AV node). With each beat there is commonly the near simultaneous appearance of R and then P wave on the VEGM and AEGM respectively. The rate of tachycardia may be anywhere between 100 to just over 200 b.p.m., and is on average, in my experience, about 170 b.p.m. Thus, it can easily fall into a detection zone of the ICD when occurring in a faster variety. The onset is sudden (commonly initiating with a premature atrial contraction (PAC) that blocks in conduction down the antegrade fast AV node pathway) and BBA and 2 : 1 conduction to the ventricles may rarely occur.

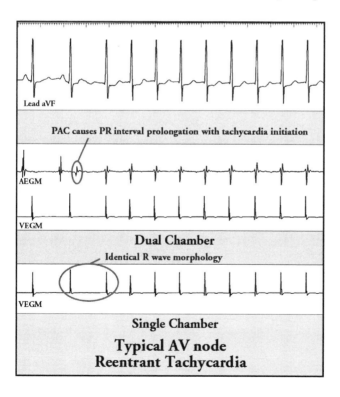

Lead aVF

PAC causes PR interval prolongation with tachycardia initiation

AEGM

VEGM

Dual Chamber

Identical R wave morphology

VEGM

Single Chamber

**Typical AV node
Reentrant Tachycardia**

11 _____ may occur when the AV node has two pathways with different conduction properties.

12 The onset of AVNRT is _____.

For the EGM interpreter the near simultaneous activation of ventricle and then atria with identical VEGM R wave morphology to that of the baseline rhythm should raise the suspicion of AVNRT. As regards the ICD interpretation of this rhythm, a discriminator such as sudden onset will not help. An ICD with ventricular morphology or width discrimination may be useful, so long as BBA does not occur. However, the sustained tachycardia rate alone, as in the previous, and subsequent SVTs, may result in the ICD treating this rhythm as a ventricular tachyarrhythmia should a sustained rate criterion be programmed on.

13 Identical tachycardia and sinus rhythm _____ _____ morphologies with near _____ activation of the ventricles, then atria, suggests AVNRT.

Atrial Flutter

Atrial flutter is commonly a right atrial reentrant rhythm characterized by "saw tooth" flutter waves in the inferior surface ECG leads and a rate of approximately 300 b.p.m. It can also originate in the left atrium and may have some variability in rate, i.e. about 240–320 b.p.m. Conduction to the ventricles in all varieties can commonly be 2 : 1 (about 150 b.p.m.). Ventricular conduction, however, may be variable and as great as 1 : 1! Thus, this can initiate a tachycardia detection by the ICD for the rapidly conducted forms.

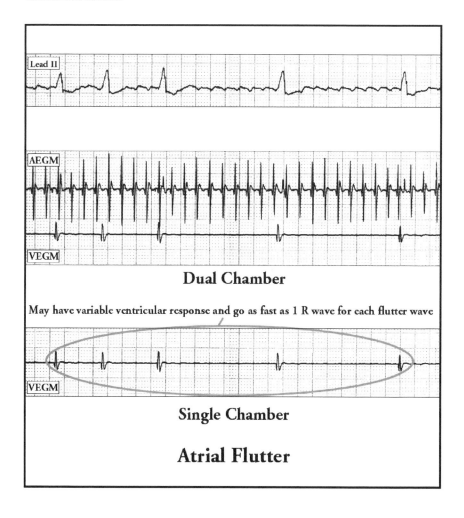

Lead II

AEGM

VEGM

Dual Chamber

May have variable ventricular response and go as fast as 1 R wave for each flutter wave

VEGM

Single Chamber

Atrial Flutter

14 The rate of atrial flutter waves may fall between about _____ b.p.m.

15 Atrial flutter may have _____ and up to _____ conduction to the ventricles.

The ICD will typically register # P waves > # R waves in this rhythm. When recorded by the ICD these events are characterized by a VEGM R wave morphology the same during tachycardia as that during baseline rhythm, so long as BBA is not present during tachycardia. A ventricular morphology or width discriminator may be helpful to limit delivery of therapy for atrial flutter with rapid conduction, should the ICD have such a function. As mentioned earlier, it is possible for a ventricular tachyarrhythmia to coexist during atrial flutter. Thus to err on the side of caution therapy may be delivered by the ICD to protect against such an instance, particularly if a discriminator function is not active.

16 When there is NOT a concurrent ventricular tachyarrhythmia, an ICD will register # P waves _____ # R waves during atrial flutter.

17 A supraventricular and ventricular tachyarrhythmia may _____.

Atrial Fibrillation

Atrial fibrillation (AF) is the most common cardiac arrhythmia and is characterized by rapid chaotic electrical activation of the atria and an irregularly irregular ventricular conduction pattern. The mean rate of ventricular conduction may approach 180 b.p.m., and as such may enter the ICD detection zones. It commonly occurs paroxysmally, and is one of the more frequently encountered SVTs leading to inappropriate ICD therapy. Transient BBA may occur, particularly with a short R–R interval that follows a longer R–R interval (Ashmann's phenomenon). Otherwise, the VEGM R wave morphology remains the same during AF as that during normal sinus rhythm.

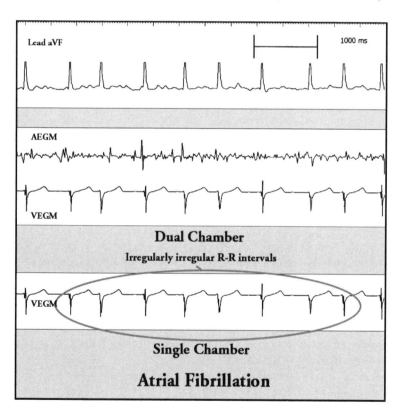

18 The hallmark of AF on the AEGM is _____ and _____ atrial electrical activation.

19 Transient BBA during AF is commonly seen due to _____ phenomenon.

A "stability" function uses the irregularly irregular nature of the rhythm to help the ICD differentiate a rapidly conducted AF from VT (VT R–R cycle lengths typically do not vary much). Some VTs though can have some irregularity in their rate, and the ventricular response in AF can sometimes appear less irregular. Ventricular morphology discrimination can take advantage of the same R wave VEGM morphology during AF as that during tachycardia, again absent the onset of BBA with tachycardia. As far as the EGM interpreter is concerned an irregularly irregular ventricular rhythm should immediately make one think of AF. Add in an identical VEGM morphology during tachycardia to that of baseline rhythm and the diagnosis of AF is made extremely likely. One would not even necessarily have to see an AEGM.

VT can coexist with AF (see below). A giveaway to the interpreter that VT may be present is a completely regular fast ventricular rhythm whose morphology is unlike that during baseline rhythm.

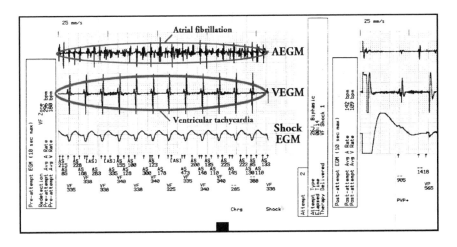

20 A _____ discriminator is frequently helpful for differentiating AF with a fast ventricular response from VT.

21 An irregularly irregular VEGM R wave pattern should suggest a rhythm of _____.

Ventricular Tachycardia

VT occurs when a ventricular focus or circuit independently discharges at an elevated rate (i.e. anywhere from 110–250 b.p.m.). Its onset is typically sudden and some instability in rate and R wave morphology may occur. By common convention it is referred to as "sustained" when it lasts ≥ 30 seconds or causes significant hemodynamic consequence and/or symptoms in spite of a shorter duration. The term "non-sustained" VT is usually used to describe three or more consecutive fast ventricular beats that do not otherwise meet the criteria for being sustained.

During VT the atria may act independently or not be activated retrogradely in a 1 : 1 fashion. Absent a fast concurrent SVT, the number of detected R waves is greater than the number of P waves in a dual chamber ICD. When this occurs it is one of the easier rhythms for the EGM interpreter and ICD to recognize as truly being VT.

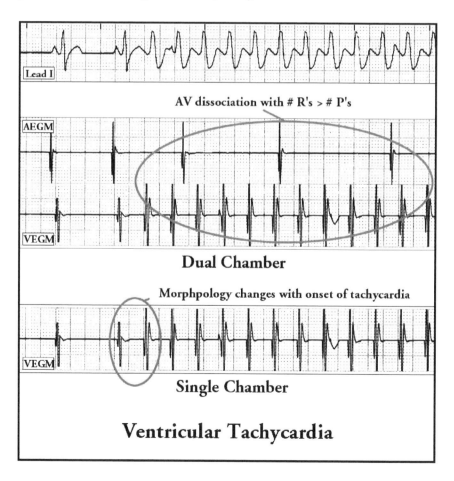

On the other hand retrograde conduction to the atria in a 1 : 1 fashion can occur during VT. This becomes more difficult for both the ICD and the EGM interpreter to recognize as being VT vs. SVT with 1 : 1 conduction to the ventricles. Should the onset of such a rhythm be recorded by a dual chamber ICD one may commonly note the initiation of the tachycardia by a ventricular beat. This may make the diagnosis of VT more likely, although some SVTs can be initiated following a premature ventricular beat that conducts retrogradely to the atria.

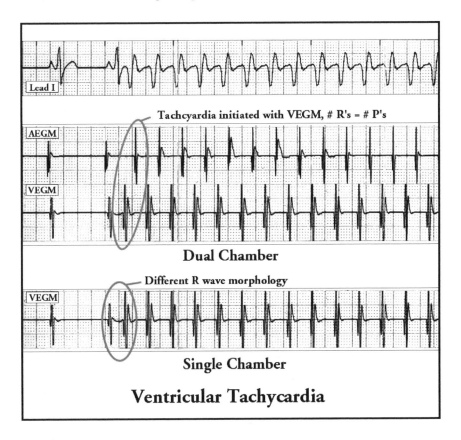

During VT a change in the VEGM R wave morphology and far-field R wave width vs. that in baseline rhythm is often noted in both single and dual chamber ICDs. Thus a morphology or width discriminator may be of use to differentiate SVT from VT. In some patients, though, the R wave morphology may look remarkably the same in VT and in the baseline rhythm.

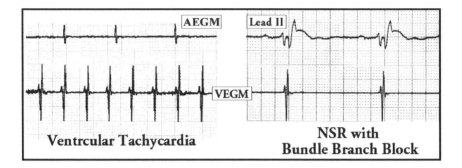

Some devices have the ability to record an additional signal between the can and a shocking coil, which can mimic a surface ECG lead. This can also aid the interpreter in the troubleshooting process, particularly when dealing with a single chamber ICD.

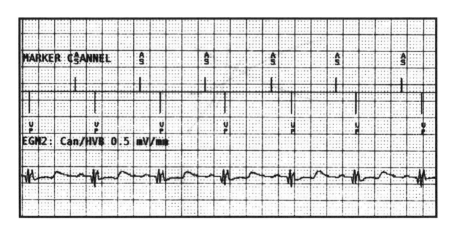

Ventricular Fibrillation

VF is characterized by the rapid chaotic firing of numerous ventricular foci that produces an ineffective cardiac output. When sustained it is deadly if not promptly treated. It may occur spontaneously or occasionally as a result of deteriorating VT. It appears on the VEGM as ventricular complexes widely variable in amplitude and morphology and is easily recognizable by both the ICD and EGM interpreter. During VF the atrial rhythm may act independently or appear in an irregularly irregular retrograde conduction pattern.

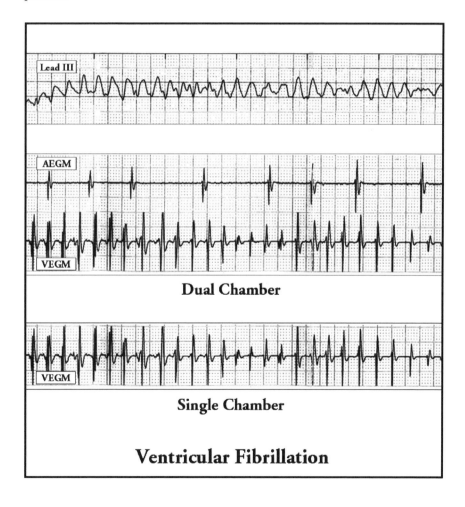

Summary

It can sometimes be extremely difficult for both an ICD and an EGM interpreter to correctly differentiate an SVT from VT when analyzing intracardiac EGMs. This may be even more problematic for single chamber ICDs where only the shock and VEGMs are available. Comparing a patient's baseline R wave morphology to that during an arrhythmic event, noting the relationship of the P waves on the AEGM to the R waves on the VEGM when both are present, and capturing the arrhythmia onset may greatly enhance the ability to correctly attach the proper diagnosis. By doing so optimal programming may be facilitated to minimize inappropriate shocks for SVT while allowing appropriate therapies for VT to be delivered.

CHAPTER 8

The Therapies

Ventricular tachyarrhythmia therapy in an ICD may be programmed for each zone of detection. For arrhythmias detected in the VF zone this occurs in the form of defibrillation. Shocks to terminate tachycardias in this zone may occur regardless of the timing in the cardiac cycle, and up to a maximum of 25–42 J stored energy in contemporary devices. Some ICD models may deliver up to eight shocks per arrhythmia episode.

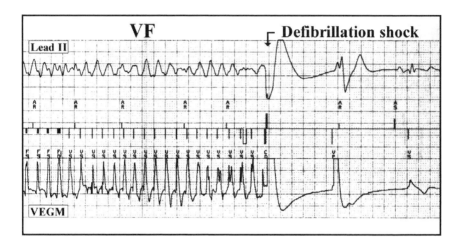

1 The timing of a defibrillation shock _____ necessarily delivered with regard to the point in time of the cardiac cycle.

2 Depending on the ICD model, it may store upwards of _____ of energy for a single charge sequence.

Initial therapy for an episode detected in a VT zone can include overdrive anti-tachycardia pacing (ATP). ATP may be effective for terminating VT occurring up to around 210 b.p.m. With this form of treatment ventricular pacing is delivered in a burst at a cycle length shorter than that of the tachycardia (typically 10–20% shorter). The tachycardia may be terminated by rendering its circuit refractory at a critical point. ATP burst options include pacing at a fixed cycle length, pacing at a progressively shorter cycle length ("ramp") with each impulse, and pacing with a combination of both. The number of pacing impulses within each burst and the number of burst attempts are also programmable.

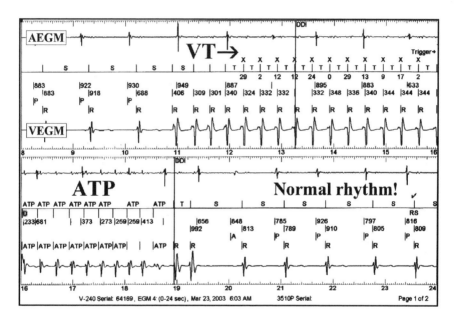

3 ATP attempts to terminate VT by pacing at a cycle length _____ than that of the tachycardia.

4 The _____ form of ATP is one in which the cycle length between each subsequent pacing impulse becomes progressively shorter.

Cardioversion is the next level of therapy brought to bear in a VT zone. Each shock is synchronized to occur with an R wave during the cardiac cycle. These shocks are always programmed to follow unsuccessful ATP therapies. As with a VF zone, multiple shocks may be administered for each episode should a tachycardia be refractory to termination. The initial shock energy is typically low (i.e. 1–5 J) and increased for each subsequent shock.

Finally, no therapy may be programmed in a VT zone. Why would one do this? The idea here is to allow the ICD to record a previously occult arrhythmia, particularly in the slowest zone of detection. This type of VT zone is commonly referred to as a "monitor zone."

5 The timing of a cardioversion shock _____ delivered with regard to the point in time of the cardiac cycle.

6 A _____ _____ may be used to detect previously unseen arrhythmias.

CHAPTER 9

ICD Pacing

Basic Pacing

Today's ICD systems have similar bradycardia pacing capabilities as a conventional pacemaker. Whether or not back-up pacing function is required for the defibrillator patient may frequently depend on the reason the ICD was implanted, and the future need for medication that may precipitate significant bradyarrhythmias. The EGMs usually do not play a significant role in helping to troubleshoot basic pacing functions. As will be seen later in this chapter, the exception to this can occur in the newer ICDs with biventricular pacing capabilities.

The New Implant

A patient without a prior history of significant bradyarrhythmias who receives an ICD for traditional indications (VT, VF, SCD prevention) will quite frequently have a pacing mode of VVI with a very slow lower rate programmed (i.e. 40 b.p.m.). Subsequently, however, some patients need higher doses of beta blockade and/or initiation of anti-arrhythmic medications. This may precipitate symptomatic bradyarrhythmias and require a change in pacing rate and mode. Because of this potential, and for the additional benefit of atrial input into tachycardia discrimination, i.e. SVT vs. VT, a dual chamber ICD system may be exclusively utilized by some physicians, unless the patient has chronic AF. This will allow a physiologic mode of pacing to be programmed, and negate the need of a second surgery to implant an atrial pacing lead and upgrade to a dual chamber ICD had a single chamber ICD been implanted initially. Other physicians may choose to use a single chamber ICD initially, as the system is easier to implant, and a significant amount of back-up bradycardia pacing may not be needed in the future in some patients.

1 ICD patients without any significant bradyarrhythmias will frequently have a _____ pacing mode with a _____ lower rate programmed.

2 Medications may _____ symptomatic bradyarrhythmias.

The Upgrade from Prior Pacemaker

Patients with an existing pacemaker who undergo removal and implantation of an ICD obviously require bradycardia pacing back-up. The mode of pacing is up to the implanting physician (i.e. VVIR vs. DDD). Many will opt for a dual chamber ICD and DDD pacing in order to maintain a physiologic mode of pacing, particularly if an atrial lead is already present and the patient does not have chronic AF. Also, DDD pacing is significantly less likely to result in the pacemaker syndrome than VVI pacing.

Patients may occasionally undergo ICD placement at a separate site from a pacemaker that is already in place. In theory one could use either device for bradycardia pacing. Simply implanting an ICD without concerning oneself with the pacemaker, however, can result in significant, and potentially deadly, results. Of most concern, the pacing output from a pacemaker may cause undersensing of VF by an ICD. This may result in delayed or complete lack of recognition of VF by the ICD (see Chapter 10)! As such, removal of any pre-existing pacemaker when upgrading to an ICD is not an uncommon practice.

Regardless of whether the ICD is a new implant, or an upgrade from a pacemaker system, a more aggressive back-up bradycardia pacing rate/mode may be separately programmed to take effect in some ICD models in the immediate post-shock period. The reason for this is that some patients may have transient bradycardia/heart block in this period. Thus, back-up pacing would likely minimize any potential morbidity from such an occurrence. For example, a patient with a dual chamber ICD may have a pacing mode of VVI 40 b.p.m., but a post-shock mode and rate of DDD 70 b.p.m.

3 Many physicians will _____ a pre-existing pacemaker when implanting an ICD at a separate site.

4 In some ICDs a separate pacing _____ and _____ may be programmed to take effect for the immediate post-shock period.

The Implant for Congestive Heart Failure

(A.K.A. Biventricular Pacing, or Cardiac Resynchronization (CRT))

ICDs with biventricular pacing capabilities are approved for use in patients who have medically refractory congestive heart failure (CHF) on optimal therapy, a significant ventricular conduction disturbance (i.e. bundle branch block), a dilated LV, and at least a moderately depressed ejection fraction. The resynchronization of left and right ventricular contractions with biventricular pacing may result in significant improvement in CHF symptoms in these patients. Aside from CHF, though, these patients also have a significant risk for developing SCD, thus the logic behind also having defibrillator function in these patients. To accommodate the added left ventricular pacing lead CRT ICD models have an additional port in their header.

Depending on the ICD model biventricular pacing patients may be prone to inappropriate shocks in certain circumstances. There will be more on this phenomenon shortly. Also, it may be difficult in some patients to determine ventricular capture thresholds. Before addressing these issues, however, biventricular programming basics need to be explained.

Many patients receiving a biventricular ICD do not have any significant bradyarrhythmias or chronotropic incompetence. Thus, for those patients without chronic AF, it is very common to program a mode of DDD or VDD with a slow lower rate, i.e. 40 b.p.m. Some patients, especially those being upgraded from a pacemaker, may have bradyarrhythmias and/or chronotropic incompetence and require a DDDR mode with a more substantial lower rate. The key in all of these patients is to maintain biventricular pacing 100% of the time rather than allowing for native ventricular conduction to occur. This is done by programming a short AV delay whose value depends on the magnitude of the patient's underlying conduction disturbance and the need for atrial pacing (about 90–150 ms; the optimal AV delay may be different for each patient and guided by non-invasive hemodynamic measurements).

5 Patients without chronic AF that receive a CRT ICD will frequently have a pacing mode of _____ or _____ with a _____ lower rate programmed.

6 It is important to maintain biventricular pacing _____ of the time.

Programmed upper rate limits in these patients should optimally be very generous, about 140+ b.p.m., and not the typical 120 b.p.m. that is nominal. Why? When the native atrial rate surpasses the upper rate limit of the device the timing of a potential ventricular pacing event cannot violate the upper rate parameters. This may result in native atrio-ventricular conduction, which defeats the primary indication of the implant, and may cause a phenomenon called "ventricular double counting" (see below). The post-ventricular atrial refractory period (PVARP) may need to be shortened, and post-premature ventricular contraction PVARP extension programmed off. These are both parameters that can result in a normal P wave not being sensed and allow native ventricular conduction to occur. In particular these parameters may facilitate non-sensed P waves of a continuous nature during sinus tachycardia (PVARP "lock-out").

Although it has not been extensively studied at present, some patients with chronic AF may receive CRT ICD devices. In these patients the mode is preferably VVIR. Again, since the goal is to pace the ventricles 100% of the time, native conduction to the ventricles in AF needs to be prevented. This is accomplished by providing an adequate lower and upper rate, and utilizing adjunctive AV nodal blocking medicines when needed. In more extreme circumstances the AV node may need to be ablated when medical management cannot control a rapid ventricular response in AF.

7 Typical CRT ICD pacing parameters in a dual chamber mode include a relatively _____ AV delay and _____ upper rate limit.

8 The preferable pacing mode in a CRT ICD patient with chronic AF is _____.

Ventricular Double Counting

There are biventricular ICD models that utilize sensing from both the right and left ventricular leads for tachyarrhythmia detection. In such an ICD, an R wave may be sensed as two separate ventricular events ("double counted") because the native conduction delay between the ventricular leads is so significant. Not all patients with such a device will double count. In those that do, double counting each R wave can lead to an inappropriate detection in a tachyarrhythmia zone of the ICD and delivery of therapy. For a dual chamber pacing mode this can occur for any atrial rhythm that conducts to the ventricles above the upper rate limit.

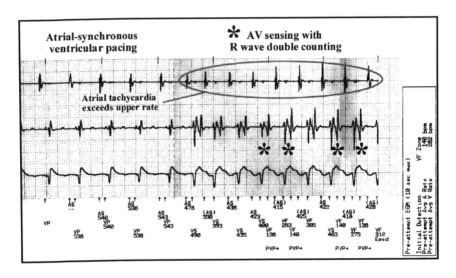

9 _____ _____ is a phenomenon that may occur in certain CRT ICDs when each QRS complex is sensed by the left ventricular and right ventricular leads as separate events.

In a VVIR mode double counting each R wave could theoretically occur when the sensor indicated pacing rate is surpassed by ventricular conduction. Therefore, it is extremely important to perform all maneuvers that minimize the likelihood of losing ventricular capture over the expected range of normal heart rates. Again, this includes the use of drugs to control the native ventricular response in AF, and potentially the use of AV node ablation when drugs fail to accomplish the desired effect.

Biventricular pacing using a standard ICD (non-CRT ICD) may also be accomplished by plugging the rate/sensing portion of a right ventricular lead and the left ventricular lead into a "Y adaptor." The single end of the adaptor is then plugged into the single ventricular rate/sensing port of the standard ICD. By electrically tying both ventricular leads together the phenomenon of double counting each R wave can also occur.

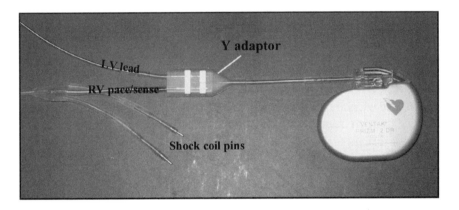

10 Controlling the _____ ventricular response is crucial for maintaining biventricular capture in patients in chronic AF.

11 A standard ICD can be used for biventricular pacing when a _____ adaptor connects a left ventricular and right ventricular pacing lead.

A unique method of biventricular pacing in patients with chronic AF can be accomplished utilizing a standard dual chamber ICD and a bipolar endocardial left ventricular pacing lead. The left ventricular lead may be plugged into the atrial lead port and the right ventricular lead plugged into its normal position in the header. The mode may then be programmed DVIR with a VERY short AV delay (i.e. 10 ms) commonly used. Because there is no "atrial sensing" (left ventricular sensing) in the DVIR mode, double counting each QRS complex from two separate ventricular leads cannot occur.

The newer generation of Medtronic and Guidant CRT ICDs that are currently approved for clinical use do not utilize sensing from the left ventricular lead for tachyarrhythmia detection, and are therefore immune to double counting because of sensing by two separate ventricular leads.

Determination of Ventricular Pacing Thresholds

The thresholds of right and left ventricular pacing leads can be difficult to assess in ICDs that do not have separate programmability for each output. This is because the morphology change of the QRS complex on a single surface ECG rhythm strip can be very subtle when capture is lost in a ventricular chamber. Also, since many of the patients for which a CRT device has been implanted have a native left bundle branch block (LBBB) pattern on their surface ECG, the RV capture and native QRS complexes can look remarkably similar.

12 _____ generation CRT ICDs are immune to double counting by not utilizing _____ ventricular sensing for tachyarrhythmia detection.

13 Ventricular pacing threshold determination may be _____ in a CRT ICD.

14 Right ventricular pacing produces a _____ pattern QRS complex.

The VEGM, by contrast, can show dramatic differences in the R wave morphology, even when a surface ECG lead does not. When combined with surface electrocardiography the task of threshold determination may be greatly simplified.

One of the keys to understanding ventricular capture thresholds in CRT ICDs is to first appreciate how a QRS complex should appear on a surface ECG when one, both or neither ventricular chamber is captured with pacing. One could potentially utilize a 12-lead ECG for this analysis. This can be impractical. Surface lead I by itself, however, may be very useful for capture determination. The predominant QRS deflection during native LBBB or right ventricular pacing (i.e. pacing-induced LBBB) in lead I typically is a wide positive complex of generous amplitude.

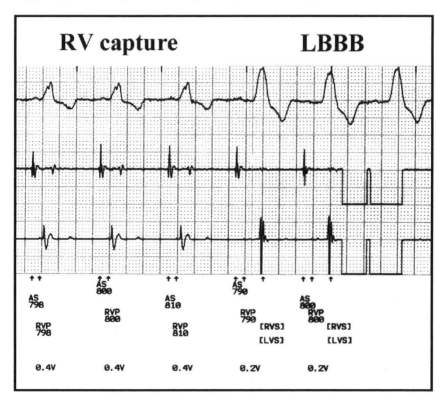

15 The _____ can be of great assistance to a surface ECG lead when determining ventricular pacing thresholds in a CRT ICD.

16 In surface lead I the QRS deflection during right ventricular pacing or native LBBB is typically a wide _____ complex of generous amplitude.

With biventricular and left ventricular capture the QRS rather typically appears as a predominantly negative complex in surface lead I.* Occasionally the biventricular capture complex will have a qR appearance (i.e. small negative and larger positive deflection) in lead I, with the positive R wave component generally not to the height and width as that seen in LBBB or right ventricular pacing.

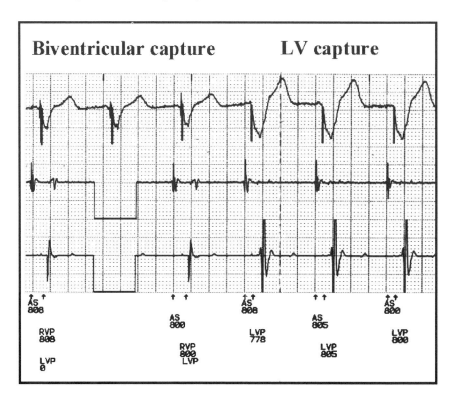

17 A typical biventricular or left ventricular paced QRS complex in surface lead I appears as a _____ complex.

18 Occasionally a biventricular paced QRS complex in surface lead I will have a larger _____ component.

---

* This assumes an apically located RV lead when considering biventricular capture. An RV lead located in a more septal location may result in a qR appearance with biventricular capture.

Thus, when progressively lowering the pacing output from above threshold in a biventricular ICD, the QRS in lead I typically goes from a negative complex (biventricular capture), to a positive complex (RV capture), to a positive complex of slightly to greatly different morphology (no capture). This assumes the most common scenario of left ventricular pacing threshold greater than the right and typical native LBBB (see next page).

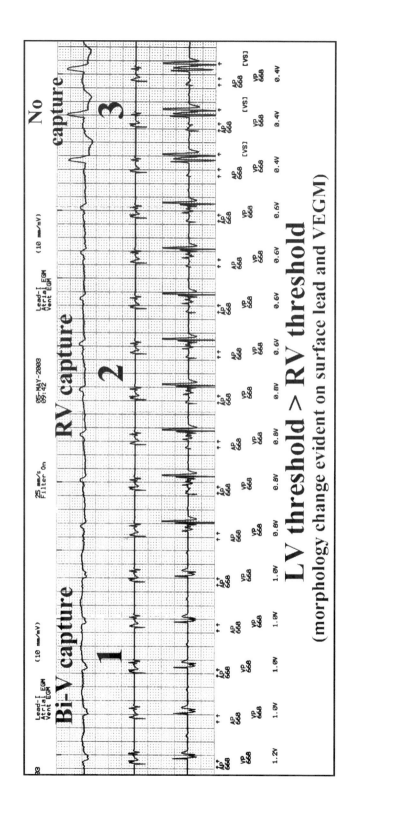

Bi-V capture · RV capture · No capture

1 **2** **3**

Lead-I EGM Atrial EGM Vent EGM (10 mm/mV)   25 mm/s Filter On   05-MAY-2003 09:42   Lead-I EGM Atrial EGM Vent EGM (10 mm/mV)

LV threshold > RV threshold

(morphology change evident on surface lead and VEGM)

Obviously the right ventricular pacing threshold can be greater than the left, rearranging the order and type of morphology change as pacing output is lowered (negative QRS, then negative QRS, and then finally positive QRS) (see next page).

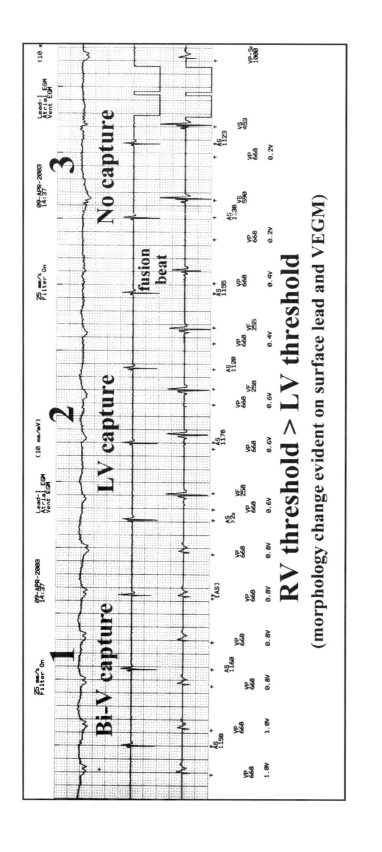

RV threshold > LV threshold

(morphology change evident on surface lead and VEGM)

Also, as mentioned earlier, there can be a less typical "qR" appearance of the surface QRS morphology with either biventricular pacing . . .

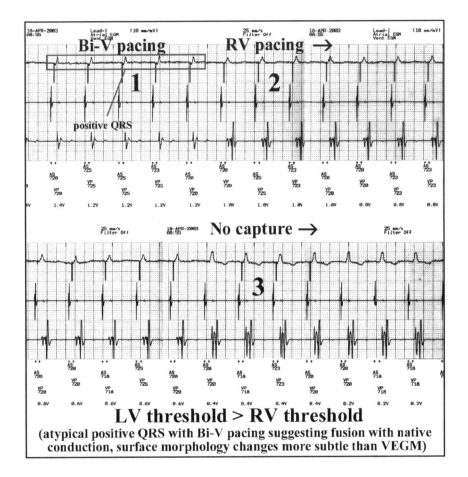

. . . and when an AV delay is not programmed short enough for complete ventricular paced pre-excitation when testing is done in a VDD or DDD mode . . .

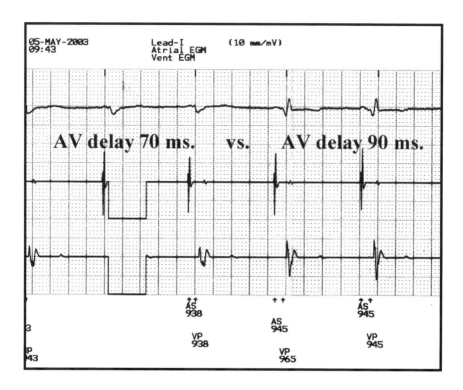

and also a predominantly negative QRS with native LBBB (possibly seen in patients with RV hypertrophy).

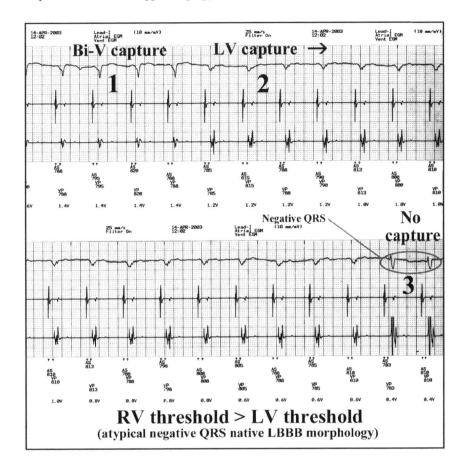

What is common with each pacing scenario, be it in a patient with LBBB or any other significant ventricular conduction delay in whom a biventricular ICD is inserted, is that there are typically three QRS morphologies to be seen during the biventricular pacing threshold test.* When less than three morphologies are seen the following conditions need to be considered:

1 the pacing threshold of one or both chambers is higher than the output the test was begun with and thus the chamber(s) was (were) never captured (if this occurs it is most commonly an elevated left ventricular pacing threshold in my experience) . . .

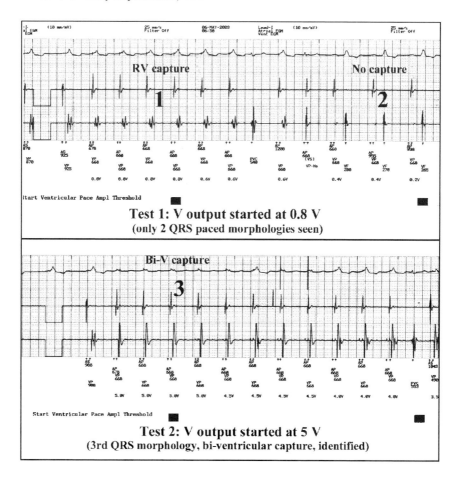

Test 1: V output started at 0.8 V
(only 2 QRS paced morphologies seen)

Test 2: V output started at 5 V
(3rd QRS morphology, bi-ventricular capture, identified)

19 _____ QRS morphologies are commonly identified during biventricular pacing threshold determination.

---

* An additional morphology may occur in the event of "anodal pacing." See pages 105–8 for further explanation.

2 the right and left ventricular pacing thresholds are identical (this should be suspected when identifying that similar acceptable thresholds were obtained at implant, there is only one paced QRS morphology seen even when starting at maximum output, and there has been no lead position change on chest radiography) . . .

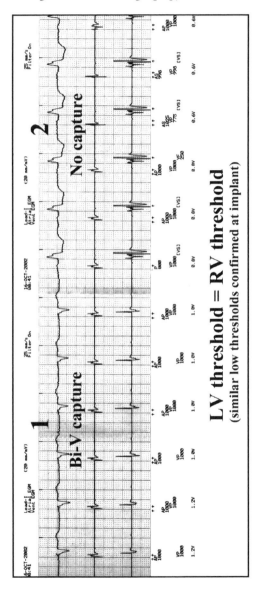

HELPFUL HINT: Lowering the constant voltage or pulse width that the test is done at may separate out seemingly equal left and right ventricular thresholds.

3 a surface ECG morphology change was subtle (that's where the VEGM morphology changes are of great assistance!),

4 there is no underlying rhythm (thus the morphologies of only biventricular capture and right or left ventricular capture are seen) or . . .

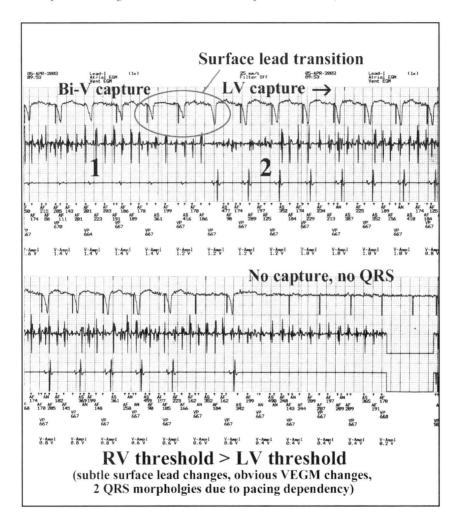

5 a threshold is less than the minimum output used during testing (temporary inhibition of all pacing can provide the non-captured QRS morphology for comparison, as can restarting the test at a lower output).

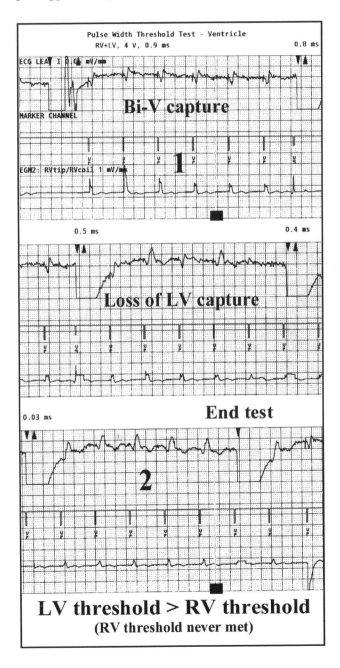

Of course with the newer generation ICDs, separate programmability and "testability" of ventricular pacing can make the task of threshold determination much easier!

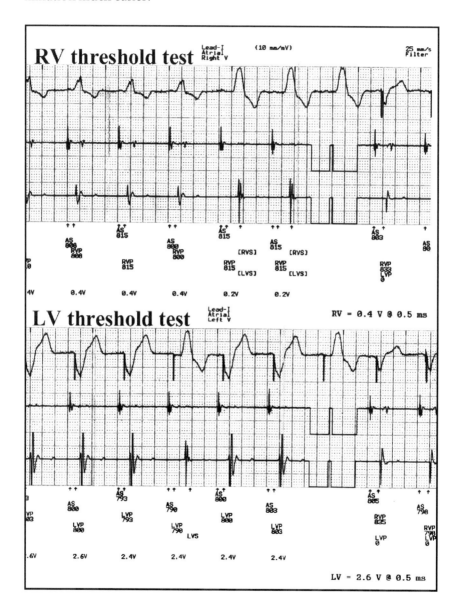

Anodal Stimulation

Some confusion during pacing threshold testing in a biventricular ICD can occur due to a phenomenon called "anodal stimulation." Anodal stimulation in a biventricular ICD refers to the capture of the RV when the left ventricular pacing stimulus is delivered in an LV tip to RV ring configuration. A large enough current density occurring at the RV ring electrode can capture the RV at this location also, particularly when a true bipolar RV defibrillator lead or bipolar pacemaker rate/sensing lead is used (smaller ring surface area, therefore higher current density than that in an integrated bipolar defibrillator lead). Anodal stimulation of the RV is more common in the implant/immediate post-implant period. When it does occur with biventricular pacing the ventricles are simultaneously captured from three different locations, LV tip, RV tip, and RV ring. Normally, capture occurs from only the LV and RV lead tips.

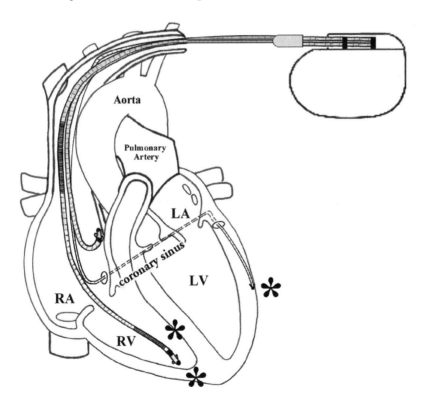

20 _____ RV capture during LV pacing can occur when a _____ pacing configuration is used.

Thus anodal stimulation may result in an additional capture morphology on the ECG during the biventricular pacing threshold test.

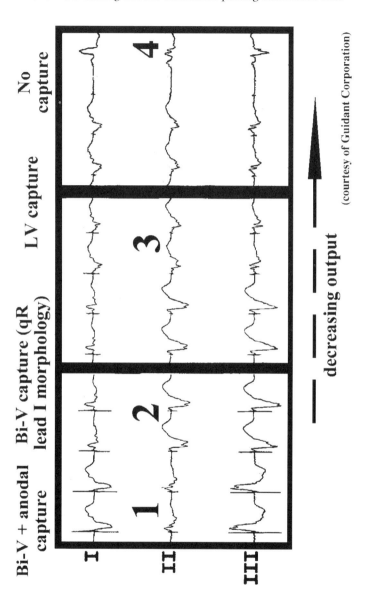

(courtesy of Guidant Corporation)

21 Anodal RV stimulation may add a _____ QRS paced morphology to a biventricular pacing threshold test.

When RV anodal capture occurs during a left ventricular only pacing threshold test a second capture morphology may be seen (see also next page).

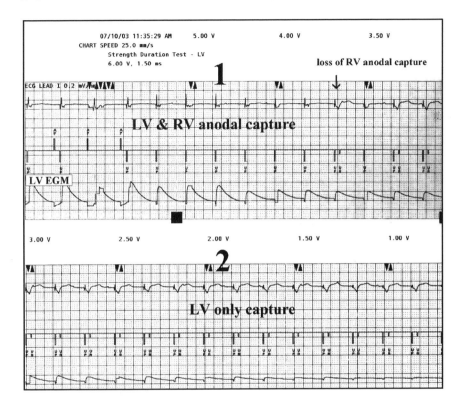

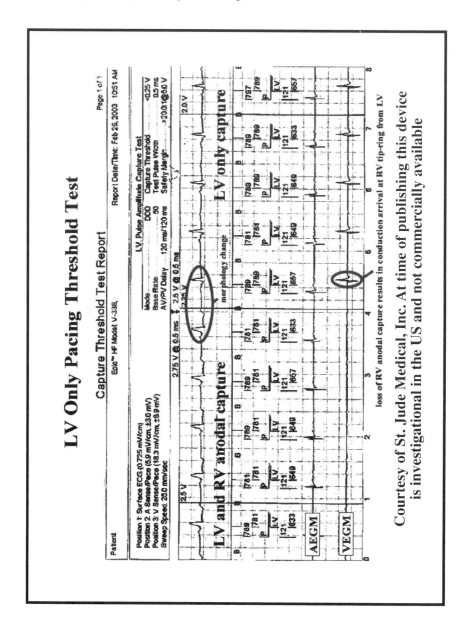

Courtesy of St. Jude Medical, Inc. At time of publishing this device is investigational in the US and not commercially available

Other than potentially causing confusion during threshold testing it is not presently known whether anodal RV capture is clinically significant.

22 A _____ QRS capture morphology may be seen during LV pacing that also captures the RV from the anode.

CHAPTER 10

Unusual ICD Situations and Alternate Applications

Inappropriate Detection of VF with Separate Pacemaker and ICD

In the past, patients who developed significant bradyarrhythmias after the insertion of an ICD that did not have pacemaker function required a permanent pacemaker implanted at a separate location. This solved the patient's bradyarrhythmia issue, but potentiated significant interactions between the pacemaker and ICD. The most important of these was the non-detection of VF by the ICD due to the pacemaker's output. Here's how.

Recall that a pacemaker has the ability to revert to an asynchronous pacing mode at a large pacing output, particularly if it thinks it is being subjected to noise. Also recall that the sensitivity levels in a pacemaker are about a factor of 10 less sensitive than that in an ICD. Were VF to occur in this setting the pacemaker might ignore it and pace the heart due to the small VF signal amplitude. The pacing spikes are of significantly larger amplitude than VF wavelets. An ICD would then have to improve its sensed signal gain or sensitivity to a generous degree, because of this disparity in size, in order to appropriately sense these wavelets. It in fact might not see them at all and remain quiescent. Obviously this interaction could be deadly.

Since the current generation ICD has full bradyarrhythmia pacing capabilities many physicians choose to simply remove an existing pacemaker, thus avoiding any potential pacemaker/ICD interaction. However should a physician wish to leave a functional pacemaker generator in place this interaction needs to be tested for. This is done by programming the pacemaker to a maximum output in an asynchronous mode (i.e. DOO, see next page) and then inducing VF. The ICD is monitored with its programmer to determine if it has detected appropriately, and an external shock applied if the ICD does not act quickly enough or at all. A significant interaction in this situation mandates that the pacemaker then be removed (in the following example the ICD action is delayed). Simply programming the pacemaker outputs down and a non-pacing mode, if available, does not guarantee that pacemaker reversion to an asynchronous noise mode at some point in time could not occur.

1 A separate pacemaker and ICD can have _____ interactions.

2 _____ detection by an ICD may not occur due to a separate pacemaker.

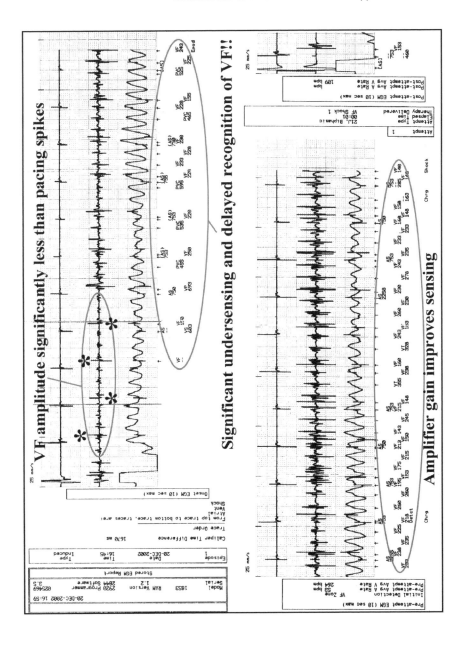

Upgrade to ICD from Pacemaker

With newer indications for ICD insertion it is becoming more common-place for patients with permanent pacemakers to have the pacemaker removed and an ICD put in its place. There are important considerations in this upgrade process. The physical position of the new ventricular defibril-lator lead with respect to the ventricular pacemaker lead is of particular concern. Why? The physical contact of both ventricular leads in proximity to the sensing elements of the defibrillator lead can cause false signals ("lead chatter") to be seen on the ICD sensing circuit and fool the ICD into think-ing a ventricular tachyarrhythmia is taking place. This can be avoided by observing that the leads are separated in space (see next page), and that there is no lead chatter on the VEGM. Positioning the ICD lead away from the pacemaker lead and in an appropriate position allowing for an adequate DFT is not without skill, however! Removal of the pacemaker lead, if feasible, would obviously make these issues moot.

3 Physical contact of a ventricular pacemaker and defibrillator lead can cause _____ _____.

4 Ensuring that ventricular pacemaker and defibrillator leads are _____ in space decrease the likelihood of lead chatter.

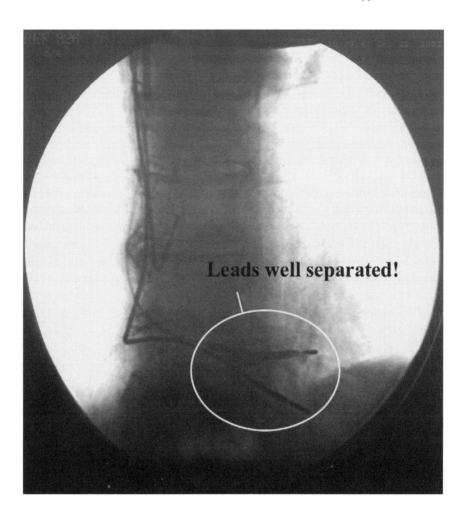

Effects of Electric Cautery

Electric cautery ("bovi") is frequently utilized during surgical procedures, including ICD placement. The cautery signal can be seen on both the atrial and ventricular sensing channels of the ICD system and may be interpreted as an atrial and ventricular tachyarrhythmia. This can initiate mode switching, inappropriate delivery of tachycardia therapies, and pacing inhibition. Because of this, ICD detection and/or therapies are (is) frequently turned off prior to surgery and restored post-operatively to avoid delivery of inappropriate shocks. Some physicians may choose to use short bursts of cautery to minimize pacing inhibition if a patient is pacing dependent. Also, some, not all, ICDs can be programmed to a temporary asynchronous pacing mode, i.e. VOO, DOO, to avoid pacing inhibition. A temporary pacing wire connected to an external pacemaker in an asynchronous pacing mode can be utilized if neither of the above options are feasible.

5 Electric cautery signal may be _____ by both atrial and ventricular leads of an ICD.

6 ICD _____ and/or _____ should be routinely turned off prior to surgery in which the use of electric cautery is planned.

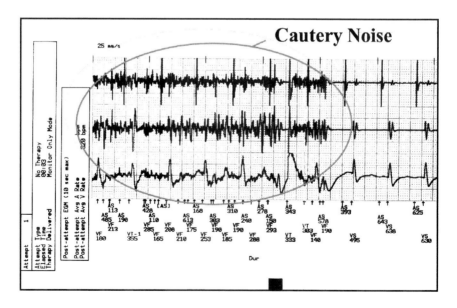

Magnet Application to ICD

The effect of magnet placement on an ICD is quite different from that on a pacemaker. For the contemporary ICD, pacing function remains unaltered. The detection of ventricular tachyarrhythmias, and thus delivery of treatment, may be turned OFF! As such, only individuals experienced with this maneuver should perform magnet application. Depending on the manufacturer, this feature may be automatic with magnet application or occur only after a programming maneuver has "enabled" a magnet effect to occur.

Why can magnet application on an ICD be useful? ICD detection frequently needs to be temporarily turned off during a surgical procedure so as to allow use of electric cautery. Also, an ICD may need to be permanently turned off when a patient is dying and resuscitation measures are no longer desired. The ICD programmer can easily perform this function, however, a programmer, or the personnel to use it, are not always readily accessible.

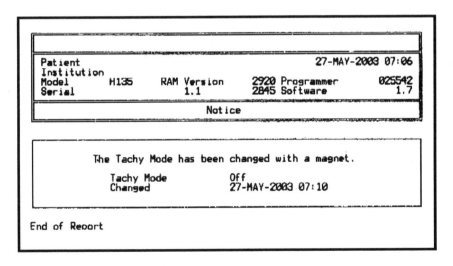

7 Magnet effects on an ICD are _____ from that on a pacemaker.

8 Magnet application on an ICD can _____ _____ tachyarrhythmia detection, and thus delivery of therapies.

Effects of Anti-Arrhythmic Drugs on ICD Function

It is not unusual for an ICD patient to require initiation of an anti-arrhythmic drug (AAD) for atrial or ventricular tachyarrhythmias. This brings into play important management issues regarding the function of the ICD system.

First, some AAD medications may cause an increase in the DFT (see below).* As such the ICD may need to be tested after the medication has been loaded or a dosage increased to ensure an adequate defibrillation safety margin. An inadequate safety margin can potentially require surgical revision of the ICD system to resolve this situation (i.e. implantation of a "high energy" ICD or addition of an SVC coil or subcutaneous patch/array).

AADs that may increase DFT	AADs that may decrease DFT
Amiodarone (oral)	Azimilide
Diltiazem (i.v.)	Dofetilide
Flecainide	Ibutilide
Lidocaine	N-acetyl procainamaide
Mexiletine	Sotalol
Moricizine	
Phenytoin	
Propranolol	
Quinidine	
Verapamil (i.v.)	

AADs, anti-arrhythmic drugs; DFT, defibrillation threshold; i.v. intravenous.

9 Depending on the specific AAD, the DFT may be _____ or _____.

* See Carnes CA, Mehdirad AA, Nelson SD. Drug and defibrillator interactions. *Pharmacotherapy* 1998; **18**: 516–25 and Carnes CA, Mehdirad AA. Effects of azimilide, acidemia, and the combination on defibrillation energy requirements. *J Cardiovasc Pharmacol* 2000; **36**: 283–7.

Second, AADs, while potentially suppressing tachyarrhythmias, have the ability to slow clinical tachycardias to a varying degree. The new tachycardia rate may fall below the programmed ICD cutoff for detection. ICD reprogramming to account for this potential effect can be very tricky, particularly if the tachycardia rate falls into a range of expected normal heart rates.

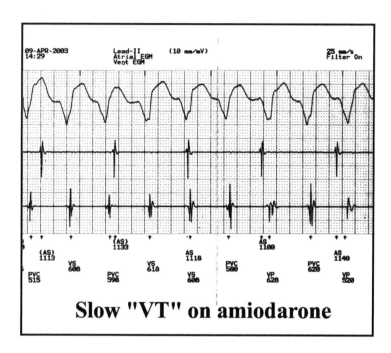

Slow "VT" on amiodarone

Class Ic AADs, namely flecainide and propafenone, may significantly increase the QRS width, and thus lead to misclassification of an arrhythmia in an ICD utilizing a width or morphology discriminator. Also, AADs may be pro-arrhythmic. This effect should be considered if arrhythmic burden increases after AAD initiation and/or new clinical tachycardias arise.

10 All AADs may _____ VT rate.

ICD Atrial Tachyarrhythmia Treatments

Newer models of ICDs may also be implanted that have additional treatment options specifically for atrial tachyarrhythmias. Therapies can include atrial overdrive ramp/burst pacing (see below), high frequency (50 Hz) burst pacing and cardioversion.

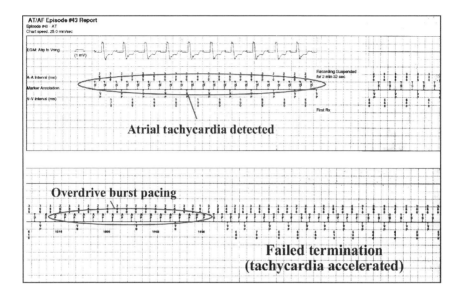

11 Some ICD models have the ability to treat atrial tachyarrhythmias with _____ and _____ therapies.

Atrial therapies, like ventricular, can be tiered based upon the atrial rate. The "benefit" of utilizing cardioversion, however, needs to be weighed against the frequency of the arrhythmia and the ability of the patient to tolerate shocks.

		Quick Look Report						**Page 2**
Parameter Summary								
Type	**Detection**		**Rx1**	**Rx2**	**Rx3**	**Rx4**	**Rx5**	**Rx6**
AF	On	222-600 bpm	50Hz(10)	Off	Off			
AT	On	188-353 bpm	Ramp(6)	Burst+(6)	50Hz(5)	Off	Off	
Patient Activated			Off					
VF	On	188-500 bpm	30 J	30 J	30 J	30 J	30 J	30 J
VT	Off							

VT/VF Discriminator: Off
SVT Criteria On: AF/Afl, Sinus Tach, 1:1 SVTs

Modes		**Rates**		**A-V Intervals**	
Mode	DDDR	Lower	70 ppm	Paced AV	180 ms
Mode Switch	On, 188 bpm	Track/Sensor	140/140 ppm	Sensed AV	150 ms

Lead Parameters	**Atrial**	**Ventricular**
Amplitude	3 V	3 V
Pulse Width	0.4 ms	0.4 ms
Sensitivity	0.3 mV	0.3 mV

Congestive Heart Failure Monitor?

Heart rate variability (HRV) is a measure of the intrinsic changes in heart rate over time. It reflects a balance between the sympathetic and parasympathetic nervous system control on heart rate. Patients with CHF may have a significantly abnormal HRV, manifested as a predominance of sympathetic tone. Some of the newest generation of ICDs with biventricular pacing therapy for CHF have the ability to collect data regarding HRV over time (see next page). These data may give an indication of biventricular pacing effect. In the future it may also be theoretically possible that these data are used to adjust medical therapy. Future research will likely shed more light on this utility.

12 Patients with _____ may have a significantly abnormal HRV.

13 _____ _____ may improve HRV in patients with CHF.

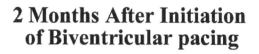

2 Months After Initiation of Biventricular pacing

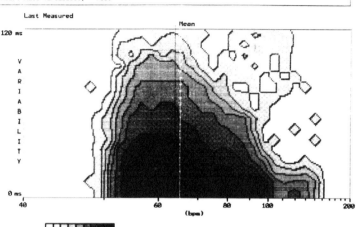

24 Hours After Initiation of Biventricular pacing

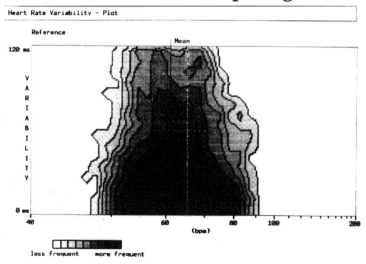

SECTION II

Case Studies

CHAPTER 11

Case Studies Part A

In this section, the goal of each case study exercise is to identify the source of the arrhythmia, SVT vs. VT. All cases are actual recordings from a dual chamber ICD. The only information given initially is the VEGM. Afterwards either the AEGM or a baseline rhythm VEGM is given for comparison. One should begin to get more comfortable with such a stepwise approach for analyzing EGMs when completing these exercises. The case studies in Chapter 12 (Part B) will begin to add more information that should provide even more "pearls" for successful rhythm assessment.

Case 1

A 71-year-old female with ejection fraction (EF) 15% has complaints of dizziness and a "racing heart." The following tracing is recorded by her ICD. What is the tachycardia?

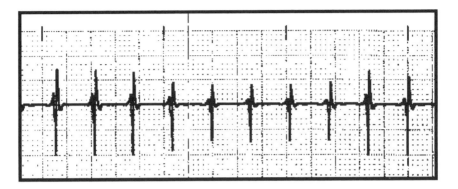

The tracing shows a regular tachycardia at about 140 b.p.m., with a single R wave morphology that has a slight change in amplitude during the tracing. The differential diagnosis is SVT vs. VT based on all of the above information.

The patient's baseline R wave morphology appears very similar, but not identical. Thus it is not clear even after this comparison what the tachycardia is, although one might be leaning towards VT given the slight difference in R wave.

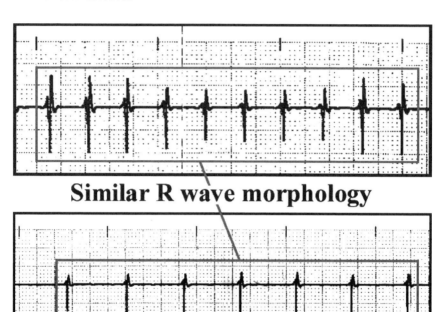

Similar R wave morphology

Baseline Rhythm

With the concurrent AEGM it becomes very clear that the tachycardia is VT (AV dissociation with # R waves > # P waves).

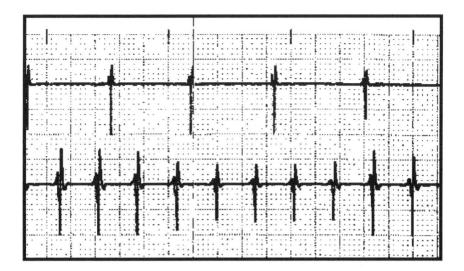

Case 2

A 33-year-old male has the following rhythm recorded by his ICD during a period in which he was engaged in an intense argument. What is the tachycardia?

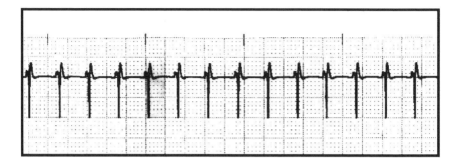

The tachycardia is regular, with one R wave morphology, and at a rate of approximately 190 b.p.m. Again the differential diagnosis remains SVT vs. VT from this information.

After the addition of the AEGM, it becomes clear that the tachycardia has a 1 : 1 association between atrium and ventricles (one P wave for every R wave). This still could be either an SVT or VT with 1 : 1 retrograde conduction.

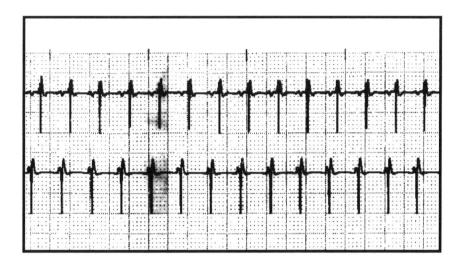

Comparing the tachycardia with his baseline sinus tachycardia (confirmed with the addition of a surface ECG) reveals identical P and R wave morphologies. Thus not only is this an SVT, but most likely a rapid sinus tachycardia.

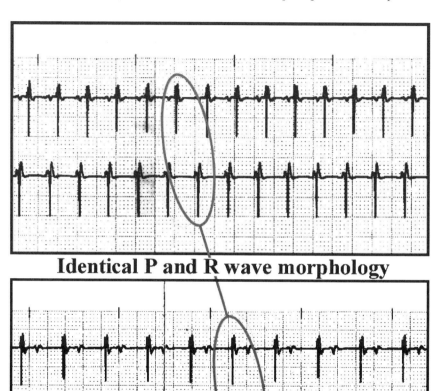

Identical P and R wave morphology

Baseline Sinus Tachycardia

Case 3

A 71-year-old female with an ICD presents for evaluation due to a complaint of "palpitations." What is the rhythm recorded by her ICD below?

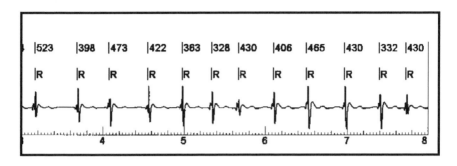

The rhythm appears to be irregularly irregular, and thus very suggestive for AF with rapid ventricular conduction. There is some variability in R wave morphology, so ventricular activity coming from multiple locations is still a possibility, as opposed to activity from a single site with normal variability.

It is obvious from the AEGM that there is AF present. A concurrent VT is less likely.

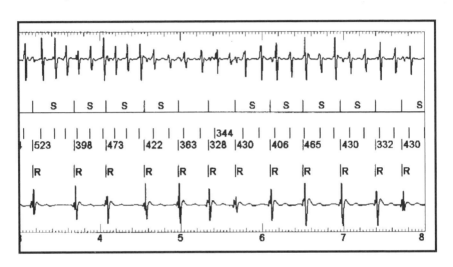

Comparing the sinus rhythm R waves to that during tachycardia reveals that she has the similar variability in R wave morphology at baseline as that during tachycardia. Thus the rhythm is most likely AF alone.

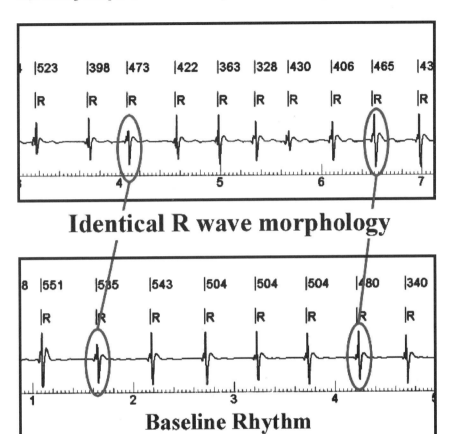

Identical R wave morphology

Baseline Rhythm

Case 4

A 51-year-old male comes to the office and has the following rhythm recorded by his ICD. What is the rhythm?

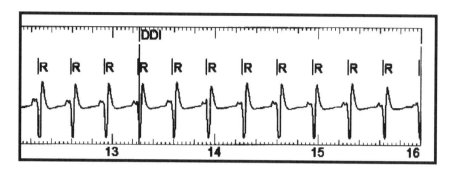

The tachycardia is regular, and at about 160 b.p.m. Again, the differential is SVT vs. VT (got the idea yet?)! Further analysis is needed to help sort this out.

The patient's R wave morphology during normal sinus rhythm reveals a completely different R wave morphology to that during tachycardia. SVT with rate-related aberrancy is still possible; however, one might likely lean towards VT as the diagnosis.

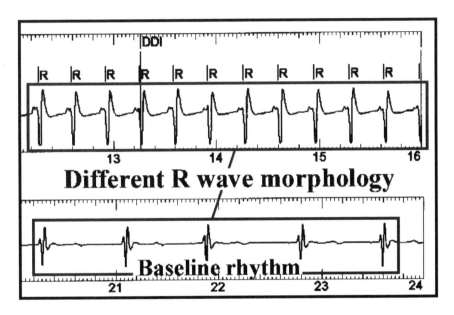

After adding back the AEGM it is obvious that there is AV dissociation with more R waves than P waves. Thus the rhythm is VT!

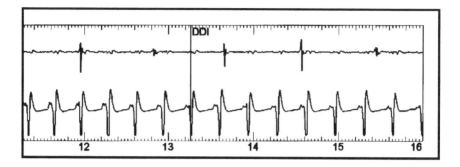

Case 5

A 47-year-old female presents for evaluation after receiving a shock from her ICD. What is the rhythm below leading up to her shock?

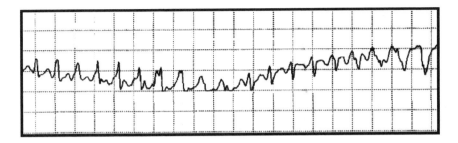

There is no differential, SVT vs. VT, here. The rhythm is VF!

CHAPTER 12

Case Studies Part B

The case studies in Chapter 11, Part A introduced a stepwise approach for identifying ICD rhythms, be it from a dual or single chamber device, based on only the AEGM and VEGM. Now in Part B, more information is included, and the manner in which the ICD handles the rhythm is brought into play. The goal of these cases is not necessarily meant to test one's knowledge, but rather to provide further exercise for developing analysis skills. ICDs from different manufacturers have functions that are particular to the device. Such functions are not emphasized here. Function may be normal or abnormal in each case.

These cases are given a rating that appears after each case number (*). As the number of stars increases, so does the difficulty of interpreting each study.

*	**Easiest**
**	**Harder**
***	**Moderately difficult**
****	**Very difficult**
*****	**Most difficult**

Case 1 (*****)

A 43-year-old female with a biventricular ICD and history of atrial tachycardia complains of receiving multiple shocks from the device without warning. You obtain the following representative EGM sequence leading up to a shock from the device. The ICD utilizes sensing from both ventricular leads for tachycardia detection.

Q What happened? (Note: The VEGM morphology is the same as that during sinus rhythm without pacing.)

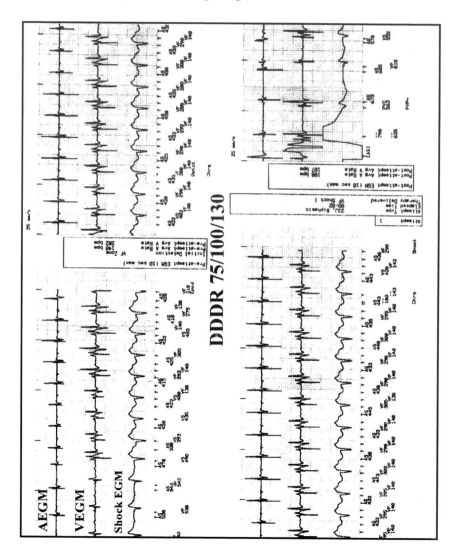

A Atrial tachycardia above upper rate that leads to ventricular double counting

Since the VEGM R wave morphology is identical during sinus rhythm and the tachycardia, this is most likely an SVT. It is likely an atrial tachycardia as the P wave morphology changes from that at the beginning of the strip, and there is a sudden onset to the rhythm. The atrial tachycardia begins faster than the upper rate limit. Because the ventricles cannot be paced at the end of the AV interval due to the upper rate limitation and each beat conducts to the ventricles, ventricular sensing then occurs. This leads to the onset of ventricular double counting (sensing the same ventricular beat by both the right and left ventricular leads). The ICD is then fooled into delivering a shock for a "rapid ventricular rhythm" (it happened to unwittingly terminate the atrial tachycardia).

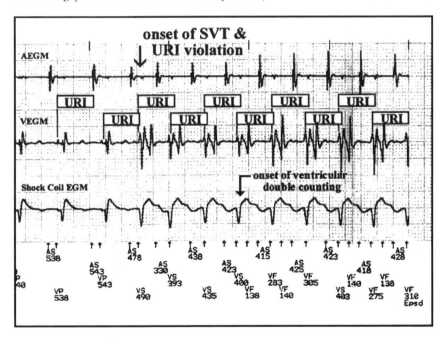

The phenomenon of transitioning from atrial synchronous ventricular pacing to atrio-ventricular sensing due to upper rate limit violation is sometimes called "pre-empted Wenckebach" upper rate response. Pre-empted Wenckebach becomes troublesome in the patient with a biventricular ICD because of the possibility of ventricular double counting.

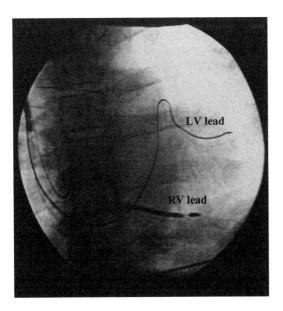

Ventricular double counting can occur when significant bundle branch block is present and a rapid atrial rhythm conducts to the ventricles, be it sinus/atrial tachycardia, AF, etc., and during VT. Due to the physical separation of the ventricular leads in space and the conduction delay between the ventricles, each ventricular lead can register its own sensed event from a single ventricular beat. The key to preventing this from happening and the ICD from being fooled is to prevent loss of ventricular pacing when possible.

Management Solution to Prevent Double Counting: (i) Provide a short enough AV interval such that ventricular pacing occurs before native AV conduction and (ii) program an adequate upper rate limit to prevent pre-empted Wenckebach. This is particularly important during a normal physiologic response causing sinus tachycardia! Obviously one would not want other SVTs to be tracked so initiation of an anti-arrhythmic medication or catheter ablation of the tachycardia focus could be considered for the above patient. Also, replacement of the ICD with one that does not utilize left ventricular sensing for tachycardia detection could be considered an option. In the future all biventricular ICDs will likely not utilize sensing from the left ventricular lead for tachycardia detection thus eliminating the possibility of ventricular double counting (so long as the lead is not "Y-adapted" to a right ventricular ICD lead).

1 Rapid _____ rhythms that conduct to the ventricles may result in a _____ _____ upper rate response.

2 Ventricular double counting may occur in a patient with a _____ pacing system and significant _____ _____ _____.

Case 2 (*)

A 62-year-old male with an ICD for symptomatic VT presents to your office after having received his first shock. He apparently was straining to have a bowel movement when the ICD fired without warning. You obtain the following EGMs for this event. The pacing and shock impedances are approximately 750 and 35 Ω respectively on multiple readings.

Q What happened?

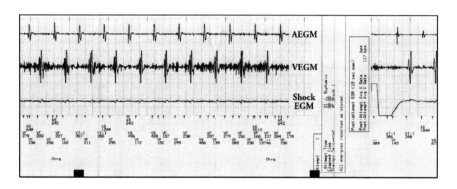

A Oversensing of muscle potentials

What is immediately evident is that there is "noise" on the VEGM being sensed in the VF zone of this device. The "noise" is actually diaphragmatic and/or abdominal muscle potentials caused by straining. The potentials continue for enough time such that the ICD detects, charges, and shocks! Such potentials were readily reproducible with straining while in the office. Why were these potentials sensed? This particular ventricular ICD lead utilizes integrated bipolar sensing making the possibility of this occurrence more likely as opposed to a lead with a true bipolar configuration.

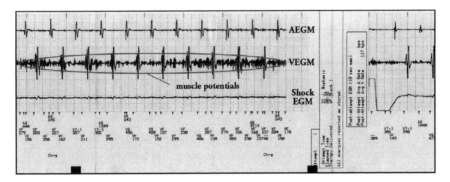

A good history greatly enhances the ability to arrive at the proper diagnosis! Had this event not occurred in this setting other explanations could have been a loose set screw on the pacing/sensing port of the ICD, or fracture of the rate sense portion of the defibrillator lead. One may have intermittently also had an increased pacing impedance though.

Management Solution: Decrease the ventricular sensitivity and have the patient strain while recording the EGMs in real time with the tachycardia therapies temporarily turned off. This may demonstrate loss of diaphragmatic/ abdominal muscle potential sensing. Decreasing the sensitivity without any other management may only be done as long as the ICD was shown not to undersense VF at that sensitivity on prior testing. If the ICD was not tested at lower sensitivities then this should be done to ensure the patient's safety. Should decreasing ventricular sensitivity not eliminate muscle potential sensing then a separate pacemaker lead may be advanced to the interventricular septum (i.e. further away from the diaphragm) and be plugged into the pacing/sensing port of the ICD. This would likely eliminate any oversensing. Removal of the ventricular integrated bipolar sensing lead and replacing with a true bipolar sensing lead is also an option.

1 Diaphragmatic muscle potential oversensing is _____ likely with a true bipolar lead than an integrated bipolar lead.

2 Diaphragmatic muscle potential oversensing may be eliminated by _____ ventricular sensitivity.

Case 3 (*)

A 24-year-old female with dilated cardiomyopathy and clinical VT (unable to pace terminate) at a rate of 150 b.p.m. receives a shock from her ICD without warning while running to catch a bus. Her ICD is configured for two zones (a 140–200 b.p.m. VT zone and ≥ 200 b.p.m. VF zone) and there are no SVT/VT discriminators programmed on. You obtain the following EGM tracings for this event as well as a real-time surface lead rhythm strip and EGMs.

Q What happened?

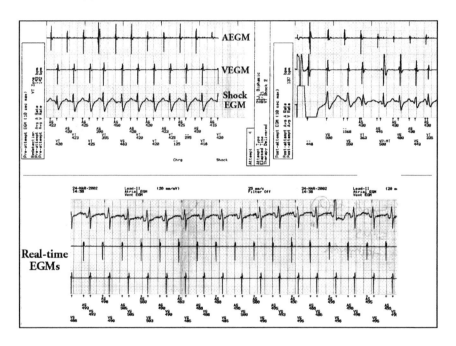

A Inappropriate shock for sinus tachycardia

The tachycardia is regular and has a 1 : 1 association between atria and ventricles. Thus the differential diagnosis is SVT vs. VT. Second, there is a shock that appears to have not affected the rhythm. Also, the AEGM and VEGM morphologies during this event and those during sinus tachycardia in your office are identical! Thus the shock during the event was for sinus tachycardia.

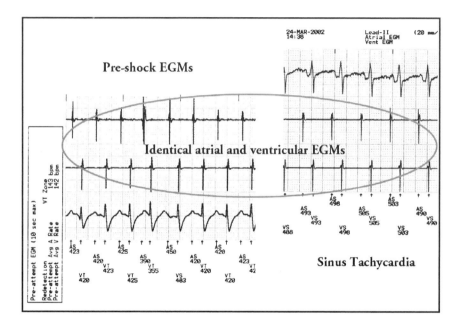

Again, the history was important here as one might expect sinus tachycardia in this setting. This is not to say, however, that VT cannot be induced with exertion!

Management Solution: Consider a discriminator such as sudden onset that may decrease the likelihood of shocking for sinus tachycardia. A ventricular morphology discriminator might also be effective for this purpose (this ICD did not have that function). Also, a physician will sometimes prescribe medication with beta-adrenergic blocking activity in an attempt to prevent the native heart rate from reaching the VT zone.

1 An unanticipated ICD shock with exertion is often suggestive of an inappropriate shock for _____ _____.

2 A _____ _____ discriminator may help minimize the likelihood of an ICD shock for sinus tachycardia.

Case 4 (*)

A 72-year-old female is undergoing determination of her DFT. She has already had two successful terminations of VF at 16 J.

Q What effect did the ICD have on the ventricular rhythm below?

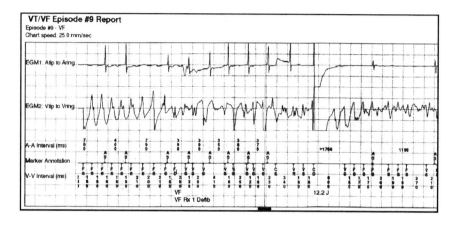

A None

The ICD failed to convert VF at 12.2 J delivered output.

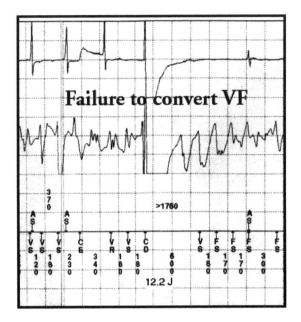

As mentioned previously, the ability to successfully convert VF is a function of dose–response, i.e. the higher the energy the more likely the rhythm will be converted. As such there is no true threshold. However programming a shock energy at least 10 J greater than that from two or more successful defibrillation conversions tends to predict future success.

Management Solution: Program shock energies in the VF zone starting at 26 J.

1 A safety margin of _____ is generally accepted as adequate for conversion of VF.

2 The likelihood of successful conversion of VF by an ICD shock is a function of _____–_____.

Case 5 (**)

A 63-year-old male with a history of a single chamber ICD for VT and ischemic cardiomyopathy (EF 10%) presents to the ER with 2 days of "not feeling right." A 12-lead ECG is obtained and shows a wide complex tachycardia with QRS morphology unlike his baseline LBBB or any typical RBBB. The ER physician believes this to be VT and calls you to evaluate the ICD for malfunction, as "it has not treated the rhythm." You obtain the following real-time VEGM during tachycardia (upper tracing) and are able to compare it to a baseline VEGM in the clinic chart (lower tracing).

Q What is the likely rhythm?

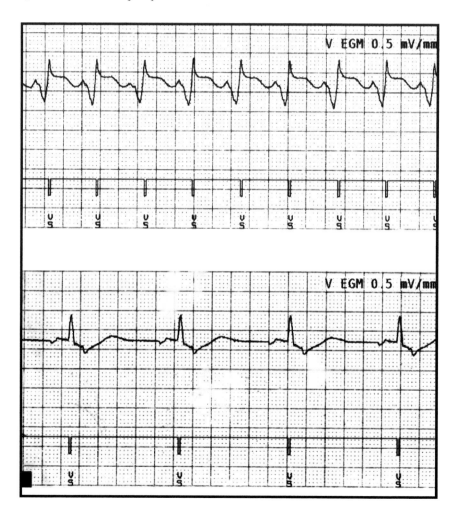

A "Slow VT" below the rate cutoff of the ICD

The tachycardia and baseline rhythm VEGMs are evidently different. Thus the differential diagnosis of the rhythm is a slow VT (more likely) or SVT with BBA different from the baseline LBBB (unusual!). VT would also be extremely favored given the history alone of heart disease with an EF of 10%. The surface ECG QRS morphology appearing unlike any typical bundle branch block favors VT. The patient's tachycardia rate and symptoms are not helpful as either an SVT or VT is capable of similar heart rates and symptom provocation.* However, atrio-ventricular dissociation could be seen on the surface ECG, and the patient's neck exam was notable for intermittent "canon A waves" (a giant jugular venous pulsation occurring when atria and ventricles contract simultaneously). VT was thus "ruled in."

Why did the ICD not treat this tachycardia? The tachycardia rate (120 b.p.m.) was below the ICD rate cutoff (subsequently determined to be 160 b.p.m. in the VT zone). This is not an uncommon reason why an ICD does not elicit treatment, and is not a malfunction of the device. This circumstance points out the importance of not delaying treatment (i.e. per advanced cardiac life-saving protocol) should an unstable patient not receive ICD device intervention.

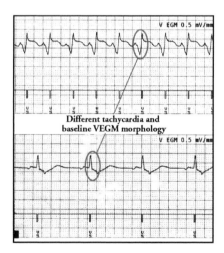

Different tachycardia and baseline VEGM morphology

---

* Very fast rates are more likely to be VT so long as the patient does not have ventricular pre-excitation.

This case is a good example of the need to incorporate as much available information as possible, history, exam, surface ECG when available, and EGMs, in order to help differentiate SVT from VT!

Management Solution: Initial management should be to terminate the arrhythmia. In this patient, after sedation was given, burst pacing through the ICD was attempted and only successful at converting the rhythm to VF, which was then successfully defibrillated. One could have also initiated an intravenous AAD given that the patient was stable.

Slow VT that is recurrent can be extremely difficult to manage especially when the patient's own sinus rate overlaps with the VT rate. The use of AAD treatment to suppress VT is one consideration. This may, however, only slow the VT further if it recurs. Utilizing a VT zone with SVT/VT discriminators that would treat the clinical arrhythmia still invites inappropriate treatment for SVT (i.e. especially sinus tachycardia), but can also be considered. As an adjunct to this approach, beta blockade to blunt sinus rate response may be attempted. Catheter ablation of the VT focus is another viable approach.

1 A VT that does not get treated by an ICD may be _____ the programmed rate cutoff for treatment.

2 An SVT and VT may each have _____ rates and symptoms associated with.

Case 6 (***)

A 52-year-old male with a history of paroxysmal AF refractory to anti-arrhythmic medicines and a dual chamber ICD implanted for VT presents to the ER because he had multiple shocks within a very short period of time. The ICD is programmed as a two-zone device: VT zone 160–200 b.p.m., 26 J, then all 31 J shocks; VF zone ≥ 200 b.p.m., all 31 J shocks. There is a stability discriminator active in the VT zone. You evaluate the ICD and obtain the following EGMs just prior to one of the shocks.

Q Was this shock appropriate?

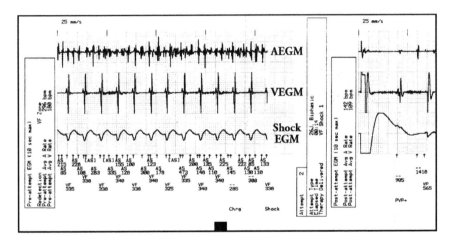

A Yes

The AEGM clearly displays AF; however, the VEGM shows a completely regular fast ventricular rhythm. Thus the patient likely had dual tachycardias, AF and VT! Both rhythms were converted by the shock.

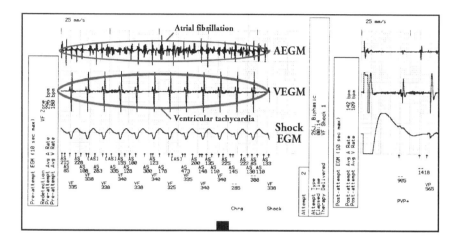

It can happen that one tachycardia leads to the initiation of a second one. This is a situation referred to as "TIT" or "tachycardia induced tachycardia." In this case further analysis of the events showed paroxysms of AF with a rapid ventricular response that became AF with VT.

Management Solution: In this case medications were initiated to prevent a rapid ventricular response during AF in hopes of preventing VT induction. Also, the initial therapies in the VT zone were reprogrammed to include anti-tachycardia pacing, low energy shocks, followed by higher energy shocks. The less noxious therapies may likely terminate slower varieties of VT with greater comfort to the patient.

1 AF and VT can occur _____.

2 Initiation of one tachycardia by another is called _____.

Case 7 (*)

A 71-year-old male with a dual chamber ICD for primary VF arrest presents due to multiple shocks from his device. It is programmed as a single zone device with an initial 24 J followed by all 30 J shocks for rates ≥ 188 b.p.m. You obtain the AEGM and VEGM surrounding one shock representative of all episodes.

Q What happened?

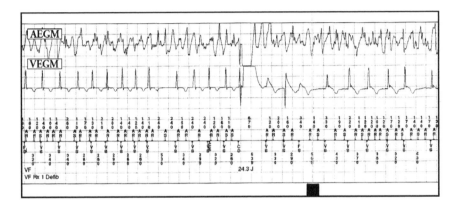

A Inappropriate shock for atrial fibrillation with rapid ventricular response

The intervals on the VEGM between ventricular complexes are irregularly irregular, and fast enough to fall into the VF detection zone of the ICD. AF is clearly seen on the AEGM. As opposed to the previous case, the AF was not converted with the ventricular shock.

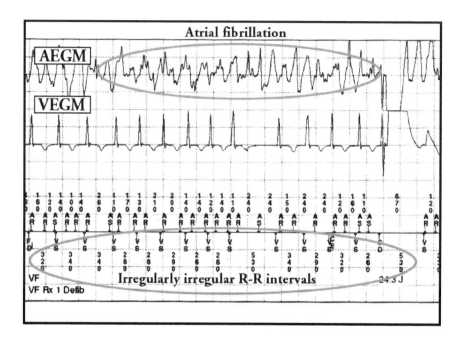

Management Solution: Reconfigure the ICD to have two zones, a VT and VF zone. Program on stability, and in this particular device (Medtronic 7274), an AF/atrial flutter discriminator in the VT zone. Also consider AV nodal blocking drugs to help prevent rapid ventricular response in AF and an AAD to suppress AF.

1 A common cause for an inappropriate shock is _____ with a rapid ventricular response.

2 A _____ discriminator may help reduce the likelihood of an ICD shock for AF.

Case 8 (****)

A 43-year-old female with dilated cardiomyopathy (EF 15%), CHF, and left bundle branch block had a biventricular ICD implanted (not Y adapted). It is programmed as a single zone device with an initial 17 J shock followed by 21 J, then all 31 J shocks for rates > 190 b.p.m. During DFT testing the following sequence of events occurs.

Q What happened?

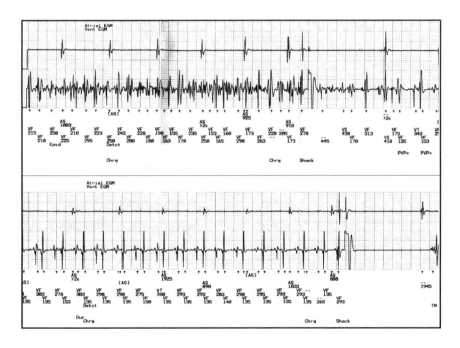

A VF organizes to VT with first shock. VT is below rate cutoff but is double counted and treated.

The initial VEGM shows VF. The initial shock does not convert this to sinus rhythm. The rhythm however then organizes after the first shock into a slow VT at a rate of 140 b.p.m. Each R wave during the VT is double counted (see marker channels) causing a redetection in the VF zone and subsequent successful conversion.

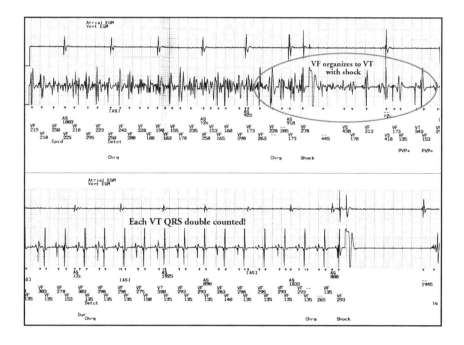

As mentioned previously some ICD models utilize left ventricular sensing in addition to right ventricular sensing for tachycardia detection. In this example the delay between left and right ventricular sensing was significant enough that each R wave during VT was double counted.

Management Solution: Since the initial shock did not convert the VF to a normal rhythm, further investigation of the DFT is appropriate so that shock energies can be programmed with an acceptable safety margin. Second it is unclear whether the VT will be clinically relevant once the first issue is taken care of. If relevant this could be troublesome as the VT will be detected in the VF zone due to the double counting, and the patient subject to higher energy shocks for a slow VT. AAD suppression could be considered, but may also further slow clinical VT if it recurs. Changing the ICD to one that does not utilize left ventricular sensing for tachycardia detection and configuring as a two-zone device (VT and VF) would solve the issue.

1 A biventricular ICD that utilizes sensing from both ventricular leads for tachycardia detection can _____ _____ VT.

2 AADs may _____ the rate of VT.

Case 9 (***)

A 20-year-old male has an ICD for a history of SCD. When playing tennis he receives a shock from the device without any warning. While in the ER for evaluation you interrogate the device and are able to analyze the VEGM surrounding the event.

Q What happened?

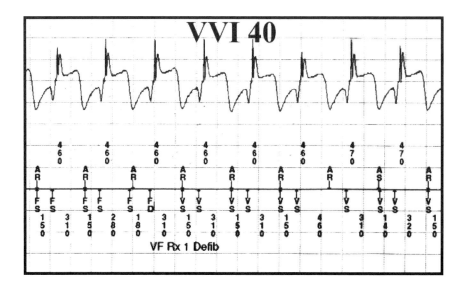

A T wave oversensing

The marker channel shows frequent T wave oversensing on the VEGM.

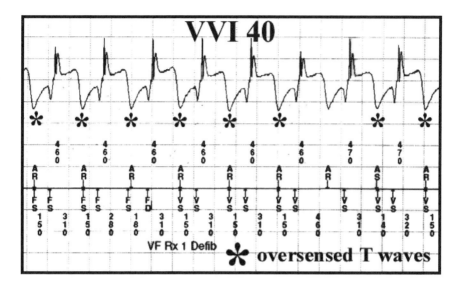

It may rarely happen that the T wave may be of sufficient amplitude on a VEGM so that it is interpreted by the implanted device as an R wave. In the instance above this resulted in the patient being inappropriately shocked for what was sinus tachycardia.

Management Solution: Decrease ventricular sensitivity without compromising VF detection. Rarely the ventricular defibrillator lead might even be repositioned to minimize the T wave amplitude on the VEGM.

1 _____ waves may be oversensed on a _____ EGM if they are of sufficient amplitude.

2 T wave oversensing can precipitate an _____ ICD shock.

Case 10 (*)

A 57-year-old female with an ICD placed for VT is undergoing programmed stimulation in the electrophysiology laboratory and the following rhythm sequence is seen.

Q What happened?

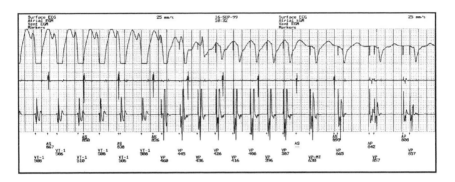

A Burst pace termination of VT

A "slow" VT (approx. 130 b.p.m.) is clearly seen on the left side of the strip. Ventricular burst pacing from the ICD is initiated, and terminates the VT.

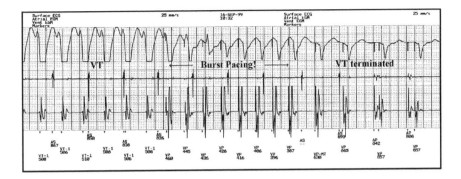

Ventricular burst pacing may be extremely effective for termination of slower varieties of VT, and should thus be considered for initial therapy when a VT zone is programmed.

Management Solution: Consider ventricular burst therapy in a VT zone.

1 VT may be terminated by _____ _____ _____.

2 Ventricular overdrive pacing may _____ VT or convert VT to VF.

Case 11 (**)

A 63-year-old male received a single chamber ICD for symptomatic VT. He comes into the office for his first follow-up and the device has recorded several events from the prior day. The tracing below is representative.

Q What happened?

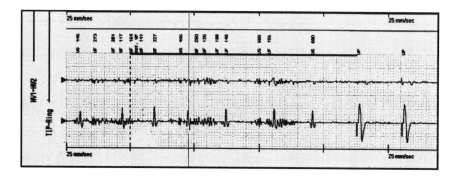

A Sensed electromagnetic interference (EMI)

There is "noise" occurring simultaneously on the shock EGM (HV1–HV2) and on the VEGM (tip-ring) that is sensed in the VF zone of the ICD. The noise represents EMI. After questioning the patient it was discovered that he had been using an industrial power drill the prior day and apparently had been holding it against his left chest.

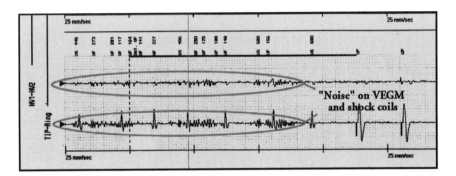

The ICD can protect the electronics from most outside electrical sources (i.e. household appliances/tools). In this case the proximity of the power drill to the ventricular lead coils and rate/sensing electrodes in the heart likely allowed the introduction of the EMI.

Management Solution: Avoid the source of EMI.

1 Non-cardiac potentials seen by an ICDs sensing circuitry may include _____ and _____ _____ _____.

2 The usual management for inappropriate shocks due to EMI is to _____ the source of EMI.

Case 12 (****)

A 75-year-old male with chronic AF/flutter and medically refractory Class IV CHF (EF 8%) with LBBB receives a dual chamber ICD with left ventricular and right ventricular leads plugged, respectively, into the atrial and ventricular ports of the ICD. It is programmed DVIR 75 p.p.m. with an AV interval of 10 ms. On the day following implant the ICD nurse evaluates pacing thresholds.

Q (a) What is seen below and (b) what chambers can be effectively sensed and paced in the DVIR pacing mode in this patient?

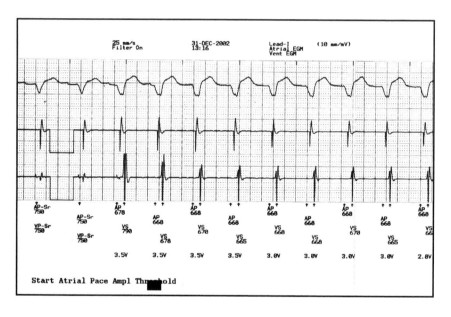

A (a) Biventricular followed by left ventricular pacing. (b) Left and right ventricular pacing, right ventricular sensing.

Biventricular pacing is essentially in effect initially (LV pacing followed 10 ms later by RV pacing with each cycle), at which time an "atrial pacing" threshold test is started. Since the LV lead is plugged into the atrial lead port of the ICD, this test is determining LV pacing threshold.

Both leads can deliver pacing due to the "D" in the DVIR mode. Only the right ventricular lead can sense given the "V" in the second position. Thus, biventricular pacing is effectively accomplished with the short AV interval, the risk of double counting is eliminated as there is no sensing from the LV lead, and the cost of the standard dual chamber ICD is significantly lowered from that of a traditional biventricular heart failure device.

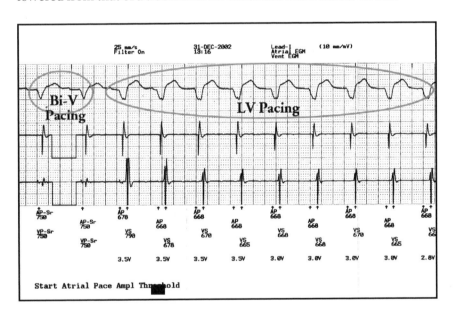

Management Solution: Normal function, therefore no changes to the ICD. Educate those who will likely encounter the individual in follow-up as to the unique manner in which the system is set up.

1 In chronic AF _____ _____ can be accomplished by plugging a LV lead into a standard ICD's _____ lead port, the RV pace/sense defibrillator lead pin into the _____ lead port and programming a short AV delay in a DVIR pacing mode.

Case 13 (***)

The same patient as in the previous case receives a shock while lying in his hospital bed. The ICD is programmed as a single zone device with all therapies being 31 J shocks and occurring at ≥ 185 b.p.m.

Q (a) What is the most likely rhythm and (b) what chamber does it originate in?

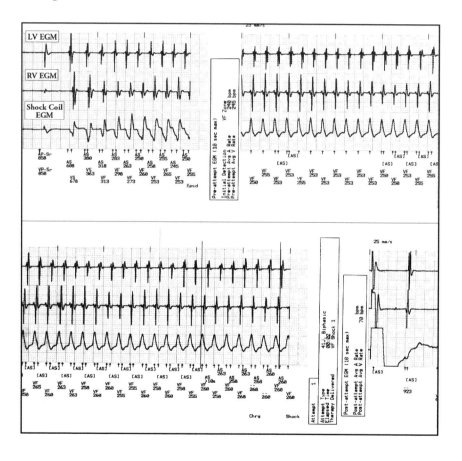

A (a) VT. (b) Left ventricle

The differential diagnosis is SVT vs. VT. The history alone of an 8% EF should suggest VT. There is a fair amount of variability to the R wave morphology in the EGMs. One may see this in VT but not likely in SVT, unless there were variable conduction defects in the bundle branches. Given the patient's baseline LBBB it would be unusual for AF/flutter to now block in the right bundle and conduct down the left (left ventricle is activated first with each tachycardia beat), and to conduct in an extremely regular fashion. Assuming VT the earliest signal seen comes from the endocardial lead over the left ventricle.

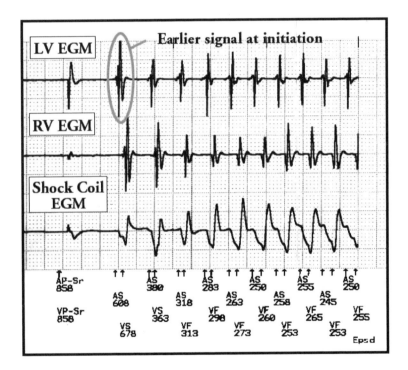

Management Solution: None necessarily needed for a single appropriate shock for fast VT.

1 A history alone of a severely depressed EF favors _____ over _____ as the cause of a regular tachycardia recorded by an ICD.

Case 14 (****)

You are the electrophysiology fellow on call and are asked to see a 58-year-old female with a history of an ICD for unclear reasons who presents to the ER because of an episode of palpitations, but no shock. You interrogate the device and find it to be programmed as a three-zone device (VT-1, 150–80 b.p.m. monitor only; VT-2, 180–200 b.p.m. 5 J, 17 J, 21 J then all 31 J shocks; VF > 200 b.p.m. all 31 J shocks). There are no SVT/VT discriminators programmed on.

You are able to correlate a stored EGM episode with the timing of the patient's symptoms. You print the episode after which the programmer malfunctions. You do not have the onset, but rather only the termination of the tachycardia. The ER physician wishes to know whether this patient needs to be admitted as the ER is full, and your attending wants to know what is going on.

Q (a) Will you be able to tell your attending with a good deal of assuredness what the episode was (i.e. SVT vs. VT)? (b) Also, if the average ventricular rate of this tachycardia was 144 b.p.m., how did it get recorded in the VT-1 zone (150–80 b.p.m.)?

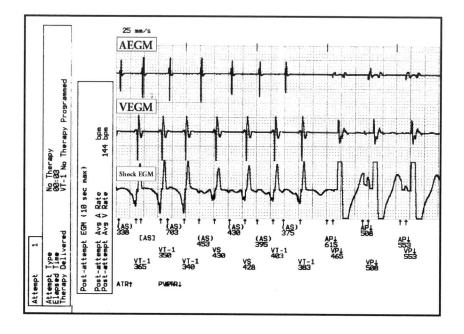

A (a) Yes

The differential diagnosis is SVT with 1 : 1 conduction to the ventricles vs. VT with 1 : 1 retrograde conduction to the atria. Because the programmer malfunctioned there is no baseline VEGM morphology to compare the tachycardia to. There are, however, some very good clues on this strip. First, the last event in the tachycardia is an R wave on the VEGM. It would be highly coincidental for this to be VT conducting 1 : 1 to the atria that decided to terminate and not conduct to the atria at the same time. Rather this is more consistent with an SVT that conducts to the ventricles and then terminates. Second, there is variability in the tachycardia cycle length. The changes in the P–P cycle length precede and predict similar changes in the R–R cycle length. This is most consistent with an SVT!

A (b) How did this tachycardia get into the VT-1 zone? There were enough cycle lengths during tachycardia short enough to satisfy "X of Y" detection criteria. Because some of the cycle lengths were longer the average rate of all fell to 144 b.p.m.

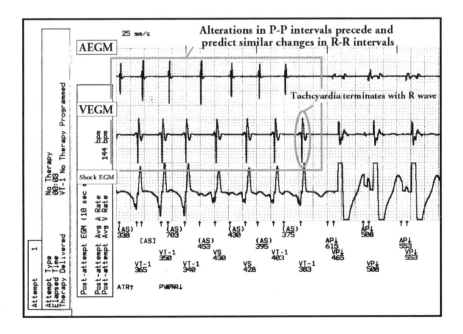

The transition points of an arrhythmia, i.e. initiation/termination/changes in cycle length, are "gold mines" in the field of cardiac electrophysiology. Their recognition and interpretation often reveal a generous amount of information regarding tachycardia mechanism.

Management Solution: A sudden onset discriminator would not likely help as both an atrial tachycardia and an VT can initiate suddenly. A morphology discriminator (not available in this device) in the VT treatment zone might be helpful. AAD treatment could be considered for frequent VT.

1 A tachycardia with 1 : 1 AV association that terminates with an R wave is more likely to be _____.

2 Alterations in the P–P cycle length during tachycardia that precede and predict similar changes in the R–R cycle length is more consistent with a _____ tachycardia.

Case 15 (**)

A 71-year-old male with chronic AF and history of a right pectoral permanent pacemaker is undergoing implant of a single chamber ICD on
the left chest due to symptomatic VT. During ICD testing the pacemaker is
programmed to VOO at 80 b.p.m. with the pacing output programmed
to 7.5 V.

Q What occurred during testing (surface lead and VEGM seen below)?

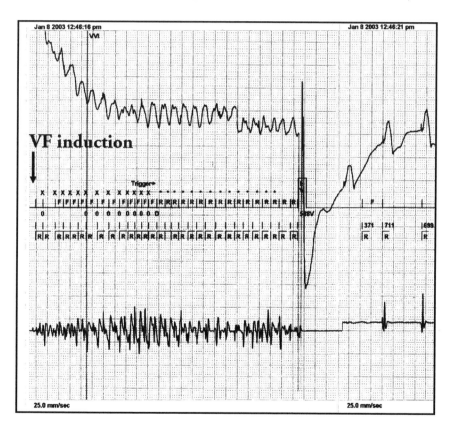

A Appropriate detection and treatment of VF despite asynchronous high
output pacing

After VF induction the asynchronous pacing spikes can be seen marching
through the surface lead strip. The pacing spikes do not have any effect on
the detection of VF as can be seen by noting the absence of undersensing
on the marker channels.

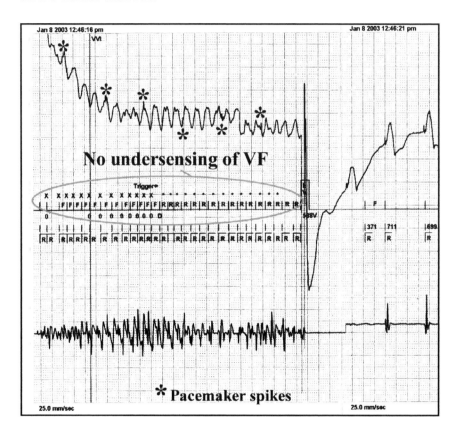

Separate pacemaker and ICD devices in the same patient are becoming
increasingly rare. This is likely so because contemporary ICDs have generous bradycardia pacing functions, and improved battery longevity.

Management Solution: Remove the pacemaker to avoid ANY potential pacemaker/ICD interaction.

1 The most significant pacemaker/ICD interaction is the _____ of VF.

2 Contemporary ICDs have essentially made the need for a separate pacemaker fairly _____.

Case 16 (∗∗∗)

You are called regarding a colleague's 73-year-old female patient who underwent insertion of an ICD for VT as well as AV node ablation secondary to
paroxysmal AF with rapid ventricular response that was refractory to medical
management. Apparently, upon arriving on the floor from the recovery
room she had complaints of lightheadedness and received multiple shocks
from the ICD. You obtained this strip that was representative of the events
leading to each of the shocks.

Q What happened?

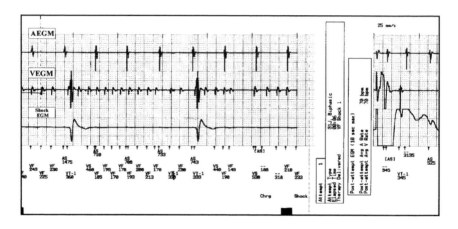

A Sensed "make and break" potentials caused by a loose set screw in the pacing/sensing ICD lead port

The most obvious finding is the low amplitude signals being sensed in the VF and VT-1 zones, and that the ventricular escape is barely 20 b.p.m. with complete heart block. The low amplitude signals are caused by a loose set screw in the pacing/sensing lead port. These potentials result because the loose set screw intermittently makes and breaks contact with the lead. These potentials also inhibit pacing. Note the lack of these potentials on the shock EGM.

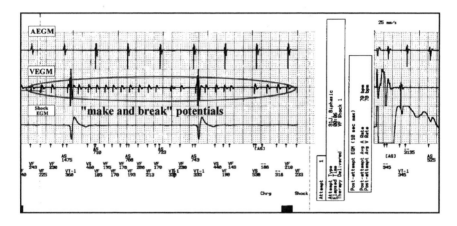

Loose set screws can essentially be avoided with the meticulous attention of the operator to place them properly.

Management Solution: (i) Advanced cardiac life support (ACLS) protocol for complete heart block (CHB) and (ii) turn off tachycardia therapies; (iii) turn on temporary pacing in a VOO mode if available; (iv) if temporary VOO pacing not available or ineffective, then continue ACLS protocol for CHB as a bridge to emergent reoperation to tighten set screw.

1 A loose set screw in the ICD's ventricular rate/sense port may result in
_____ _____ _____ potentials that can _____ pacing and precipitate inappropriate _____.

2 Close attention to proper set screw tightening will minimize the likelihood of a _____ set screw.

Case 17 (*)

An 18-year-old male with hypertrophic cardiomyopathy receives a dual chamber ICD for prevention of SCD. On the day following implant an interrogation is performed and reveals a "non-sustained tachycardia" recorded in the logbook from the prior day.

Q Is this a cause for concern?

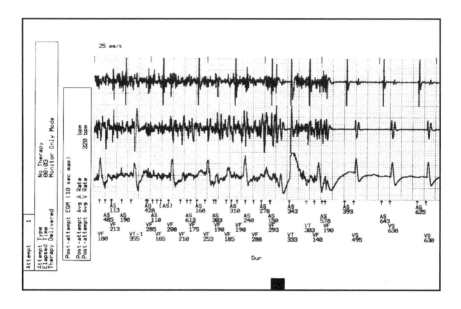

A No

The recording is "noise" from a cautery knife ("bovi") used during implant at a time when the ICD detection remained on, but the therapies were programmed off. Why could this not be due to loose set screws? One would have to have loose set screws in all leads inserted in the ICD header in order for that to happen (unheard of in my experience). Also, the noise seen in that situation would not likely occur simultaneously on each separate circuit (atrial, ventricular pace/sense, ventricular shock) as in this case.

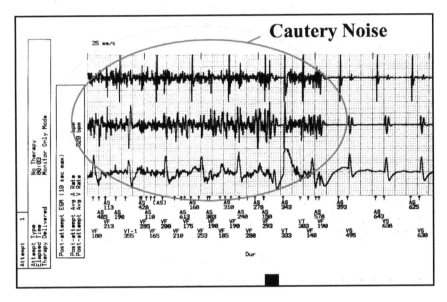

Use of a bovi is common during ICD insertion, as well as other surgical procedures in patients with ICDs already inserted. The operator needs to be aware that the signal can easily be seen by the ICD and inappropriately interpreted as a significant ventricular tachyarrhythmia, should detection remain on. If the bovi were used long enough, and detection and therapies were both programmed on, then a shock might easily occur.

Management Solution: Make sure detection and/or therapies are programmed off if use of a bovi is needed.

1 The signal from a cautery knife may be _____ by an ICD.

2 It is important to turn off ICD tachycardia _____ or _____ when utilizing a cautery knife.

Case 18 (**)

An 83-year-old male with a history of an ICD for inducible VT is admitted for sustained "racing heart" and shortness of breath. The ICD is programmed as a two-zone device with a monitor zone (no therapies) from 143–88 b.p.m., and a VF zone 3,188 b.p.m. There are no SVT/VT discriminators programmed on. While interrogating the device he appears to be in the tachycardia. The surface ECG during tachycardia (not seen here) shows a narrow QRS complex rhythm and chest radiography reveals unchanged appropriate lead positions from implant. The following EGM strip is representative of it.

Q What is the likely rhythm?

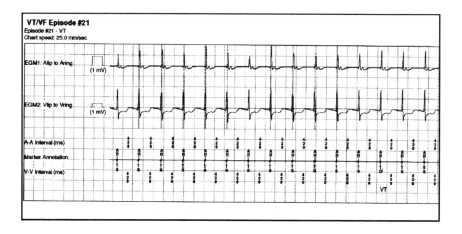

A Typical AV node reentrant tachycardia

The differential diagnosis of this regular narrow QRS complex rhythm with 1 : 1 AV relationship at such a short interval between R and P waves is essentially typical AV node reentrant tachycardia (AVNRT) vs. atrial tachycardia with a severe first degree AV block. The interval between each R wave and subsequent P wave appears fixed. An atrial or sinus tachycardia does not have this fixed relationship between R and subsequent P wave, and typically may display variation in the interval between them. Thus, from the EGMs this is most likely typical AVNRT.

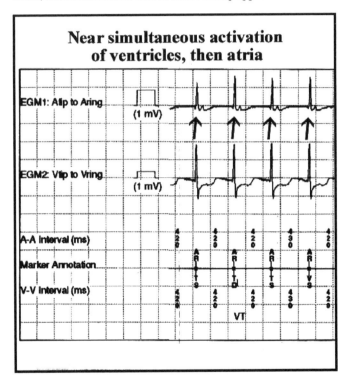

AVNRT was essentially proved by transiently burst pacing the ventricle through the ICD at a rate just faster than the tachycardia, that accelerated the tachycardia without terminating it. The electrophysiologic term used to describe this maneuver is "entrainment." The sequence of events after pacing was stopped was consistent with AVNRT.*

---

* See Knight BP, Zivin A, Souza J *et al.* A technique for the rapid diagnosis of atrial tachycardia in the electrophysiology laboratory. *J Am Coll Cardiol* 1999; **33**: 775–81 for details regarding the application of this maneuver for differentiating certain SVTs.

Management Solution: Consider increasing AV node blocking drugs vs. curative catheter ablation (this patient underwent successful ablation of the AV node slow pathway).

1 Near _____ activation of the ventricles then atria during a tachycardia is suggestive of typical AVNRT.

2 The ICD may be used as a diagnostic tool for differentiating _____ from atrial tachycardia through the use of _____.

Case 19 (****)

A 41-year-old male with severe non-ischemic dilated cardiomyopathy (EF 10%), severe first degree (400 ms PR interval) and LBBB, and medically refractory CHF receives a biventricular ICD and subsequently develops paroxysmal AF (PAF). He initially does well; however, his blood pressure limits the ability to treat the PAF, and he presents to your office in florid CHF. The following strip is obtained. The bradycardia pacing mode is DDD with lower rate of 40 p.p.m., upper rate of 150 p.p.m., and mode switching is programmed on.

Q What is wrong with this picture?

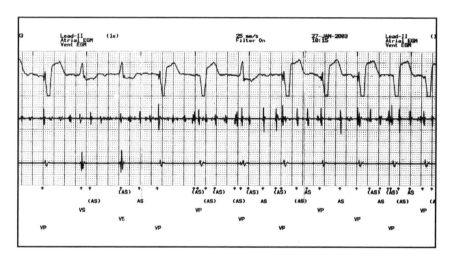

A Undersensing of AF, intermittent tracking of AF waves, no mode switching, and relatively rapid intermittent native conduction of AF waves to ventricles that inhibits biventricular pacing

Where does one start here? The AF waves are intermittently undersensed. This causes mode switching to not occur. Because of this there is tracking of the AF waves that are intermittently sensed, and at rates more rapid than one would like to have in a person with such a poorly functioning heart. Also, there is native conduction of the AF, again at rates not optimal for this patient. This intermittently inhibits biventricular pacing, which defeats the primary purpose the device was implanted.

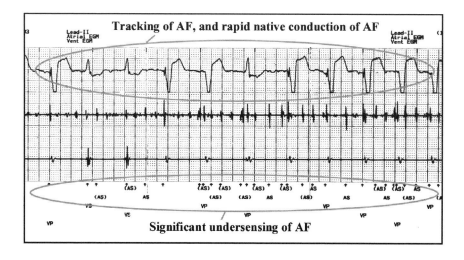

The appearance of new AF is not surprising in patients with severe cardiomyopathy.

Management Solution: (i) Admit patient for CHF management. (ii) Increase atrial sensitivity. This would hopefully improve the ability to mode switch, and eliminate tracking of AF. If this does not improve sensing in AF, VVIR pacing rather than DDD pacing may be required. (iii) Consider ablation of the patient's AV node (as was done in this patient). Ablation would prevent native ventricular conduction from inhibiting biventricular pacing. (iv) Consider the need to use an AAD (choice essentially amiodarone) and cardioverting the AF.

1 Rapidly conducted _____ may inhibit ventricular pacing in a biventricular pacing system.

2 Intermittent _____ of AF may result in the inability to mode switch and the inappropriate tracking of AF waves.

Case 20 (*)

A 65-year-old female with a history of VT and paroxysmal AF (PAF) receives a dual chamber ICD that has a morphology discriminator programmed on in a VT zone. An example of the atrial and ventricular EGMs during sinus rhythm is obtained below.

Q Will the morphology discriminator as programmed likely be helpful in this patient?

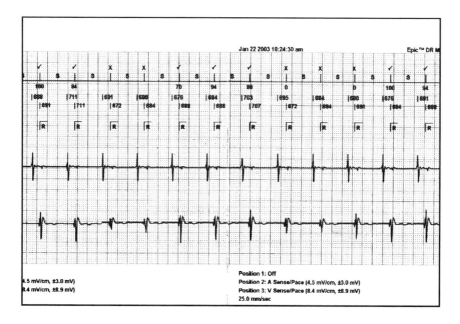

A No

There are two predominant R wave morphologies seen on the VEGM. Along with the marker channels at the top are annotations designating whether each ventricular beat did (√ **mark**) or did not (**X mark**) match the baseline R wave template. There appears an admixture of both marks, depending on which R wave morphology was seen. Thus, the ICD may not be able to confirm an SVT based on morphology discrimination.

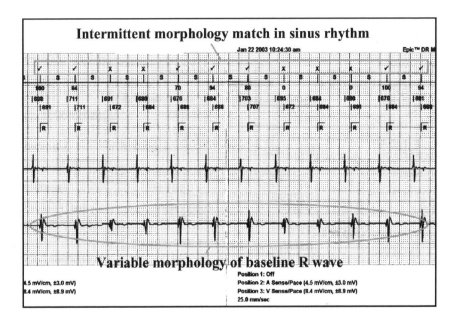

Why does this patient appear to have two different R wave morphologies? It can happen that an individual may have an intermittent conduction defect that changes the ventricular activation pattern. The orientation of the ventricular lead electrodes with respect to the heart could potentially be different depending on the time in the respiratory cycle and the RV volume. In each case the VEGM R wave morphology could change.

Management Solution: A stability discriminator in a VT zone may be helpful to minimize inappropriate shocks for PAF if the patient is prone to rapid ventricular conduction during the rhythm.

1 A morphology discriminator may be helpful for confirming a _____ tachycardia.

2 R wave morphology may change when the _____ of the ventricular defibrillator lead with respect to the heart is altered.

Case 21 (**)

A 43-year-old female is seen after receiving a shock from her ICD.

Q Is there anything unusual about the post-shock events?

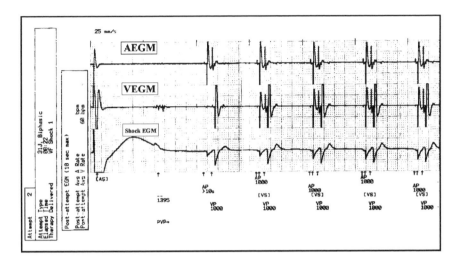

A Ventricular sensing during cross chamber blanking period

There are ventricular sensed events shortly after each atrial pacing spike, during the cross chamber blanking period. They are likely due to the atrial pacing spikes themselves. Post-shock pacing outputs are typically programmed very high to ensure capture since thresholds for pacing can be higher after a shock. The manufacturer also suggested that residual voltage from the shock could have been sensed on the ventricular channel in this period.

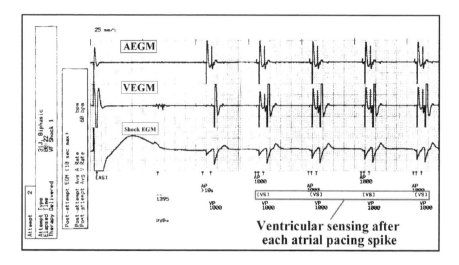

Management Solution: None needed.

1 Pacing outputs after a shock are typically programmed _____.

2 An atrial pacing spike sensed by the ventricular channel outside of the blanking period is a form of _____.

Case 22 (**)

A 69-year-old female with revascularized ischemic cardiomyopathy (EF 20%) and inducible VT (rate 200 b.p.m.) received a single chamber ICD. Two months post-implant she has an episode of syncope after a prolonged feeling of "racing heart." She does not recall getting a shock. The ICD is programmed as a single zone device with therapies occurring at ≥ 185 b.p.m. (23 J shock followed by all 31 J shocks). You find the following EGM event with appropriate sensing leading up to a successful shock ~5 seconds after detection in the VF zone. The real-time VEGM is represented below the event.

Q What likely happened?

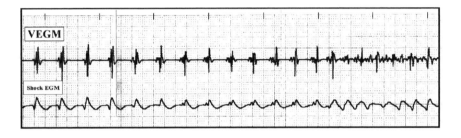

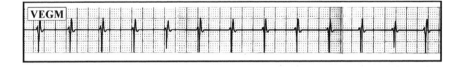

A VT below rate cutoff degenerating to VF

Initially there is a regular tachycardia at ~140 b.p.m. whose R wave morphology is different from that at baseline and thus very suggestive of VT in this setting (SVT with BBA is also possible, but probably less likely). The rate of the rhythm is below the VF zone cutoff but then enters it as the tachycardia degenerates into VF. The initial tachycardia might have caused significant hemodynamic compromise and then syncope, thus explaining the absence of a shock felt by the patient.

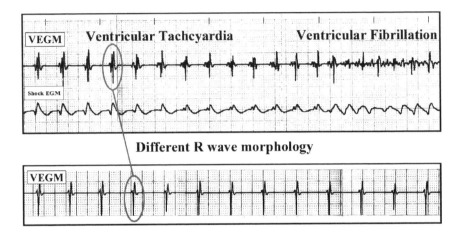

Clinical VT is commonly not as rapid as VT induced in the electrophysiology lab. In this instance the tachycardia was significantly slower. Also, it is not unusual for VT to degenerate into VF.

Management Solution: Consider empirically programming an additional VT zone (rate cutoff 130 b.p.m.) with initial therapies to include ATP, and then low energy cardioversions, followed by high energy shocks. This may terminate VT prior to hemodynamic collapse and prevent syncope. It needs to be closely watched, however, that the sinus rate does not enter this zone, so SVT/VT discriminators should be programmed on (i.e. sudden onset), and the physician may consider beta blockade medication. One might also provide the patient with an event monitor (a type of external ECG monitor) to verify the proper diagnosis of the initial arrhythmia as VT as opposed to SVT with aberrancy.

1 VT left untreated by an ICD is not uncommonly _____ the rate cutoff of therapy.

2 VT induced in the electrophysiology lab is frequently _____ than clinical VT.

Case 23 (****)

A 71-year-old female received a biventricular ICD for medically refractory Class IV CHF (EF 10%)/dilated left ventricle, and LBBB. One month post-implant she experiences multiple shocks over a few hours. The ICD is interrogated and five sustained episodes of a tachycardia terminated with shocks, as well as multiple non-sustained episodes (all identical tachycardias, see example below) are noted. The ICD is programmed as a three-zone device, VF ≥ 200 b.p.m. (all 31 J shocks), VT-2 180–200 b.p.m. (all 31 J shocks), and VT-1 150–80 b.p.m. (monitor only).

Q What is the tachycardia?

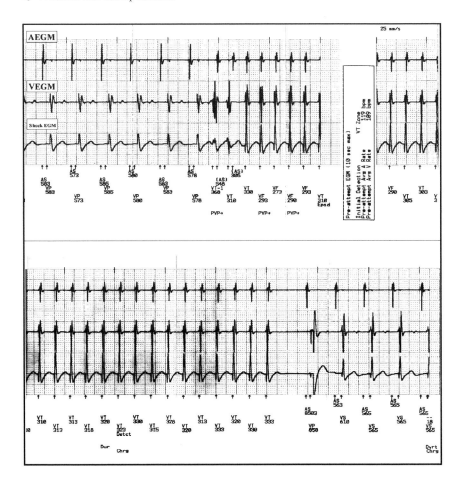

A Typical AVNRT

A tachycardia with R wave morphology identical to that in sinus rhythm and near-simultaneous activation of the ventricles, then the atria with each beat is seen. This is most likely typical AVNRT, however initiated after two PVCs that conduct retrogradely to the atria. The retrograde P waves act like PACs and initiate the rhythm.

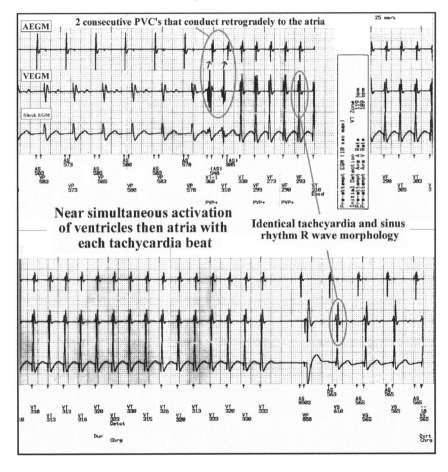

Note the difference in interval between the R waves and subsequent P waves with the PVCs (longer) and the AVNRT beats (shorter). This interval difference occurs because it physically takes longer for the electrical signal to travel to the atria from the ventricular site of origin during retrograde conduction as opposed to the signal conducting outwards from the AV node and reaching both the atria and ventricles.

Management Solution: (i) Increase AV nodal blocking drugs to prevent AVNRT. (ii) If unsuccessful or not preferred, consider curative catheter ablation. (iii) Consider reconfiguring therapies in the VT zone as was also done in this patient. It was seen that the tachycardia was terminated with a single PVC and thus might be amenable to ventricular ATP. The therapy zones were reconfigured to take advantage of the likely ability to successfully terminate breakthrough AVNRT, as well as VT, should it arise, with ATP in the VT-two zone: VT-1 150–70 (no therapies), VT-2 170–200 (ventricular burst pacing, then low energy cardioversions, followed by high energy shocks), VF ≥ 200 b.p.m. (all 31 J shocks).

```
┌─────────────────────────────────────────────────────────────────────┐
│ ┌───────────────────────────────────────────────────────────────┐   │
│ │ Patient                              28-APR-2003 13:44          │   │
│ │ Institution                                                     │   │
│ │ Model      H115    RAM Version   2920 Programmer    025780      │   │
│ │ Serial             1.2           2844 Software         3.5      │   │
│ └───────────────────────────────────────────────────────────────┘   │
│              Arrhythmia Logbook Report                                │
│                                                                       │
│ Episode Query Selections                                             │
│                                                                       │
│ Show All Episodes                                                     │
└─────────────────────────────────────────────────────────────────────┘
```

Episode	Date/Time	Type	Rate bpm / Zone	Therapy/ Duration	V > A	Stab ms	A F i b	Ons
39	18-APR-03 08:04	Spont	VT	190	ATPx1	T	6	0	25%
38	17-APR-03 23:55	Spont	VT	170	ATPx1	T	7	0	50%
37	10-APR-03 23:59	Spont	VT	180	ATPx1	T	13	0	34%
36	10-APR-03 23:59	Spont	VT	173	ATPx1	T	8	0	19%
35	06-APR-03 02:13	Spont	VT-1	169	ATPx1	T	5	0	19%
34	06-APR-03 00:20	Spont		80	Nonsustained	F	0	0	37%
33	01-APR-03 18:20	Spont			Nonsustained	-	0	-	6%
32	28-MAR-03 00:22	Spont	VT	168	ATPx1	T	29	0	34%
31	13-MAR-03 20:13	Spont	VT-1	162	No Thpy Pgmd	T	11	0	37%
30	12-FEB-03 21:53	Spont	VT-1	175	No Thpy Pgmd	T	8	0	34%
29	12-FEB-03 21:51	Spont	VT-1	115	No Thpy Pgmd	T	85	0	31%
28	12-FEB-03 19:12	Spont	VT	185	Diverted	T	9	0	31%
27	12-FEB-03 19:10	Spont	VT	182	Diverted	T	3	0	41%
26	12-FEB-03 18:47	Spont	VT	190	Diverted	T	7	0	34%
25	12-FEB-03 18:43	Spont	VT	188	Diverted	T	11	0	31%
24	12-FEB-03 18:20	Spont	VT	180	31J	T	6	0	34%
23	12-FEB-03 18:12	Spont	VT	190	Diverted	T	8	0	34%
22	12-FEB-03 18:11	Spont	VT	185	Diverted	T	8	0	34%
21	12-FEB-03 18:11	Spont	VT-1	183	No Thpy Pgmd	T	5	0	34%
20	12-FEB-03 18:08	Spont	VT-1	178	No Thpy Pgmd	T	4	0	34%
19	12-FEB-03 18:01	Spont	VT-1	130	No Thpy Pgmd	T	109	0	37%
18	12-FEB-03 18:00	Spont	VT-1	178	No Thpy Pgmd	T	4	0	41%
17	12-FEB-03 17:54	Spont	VT	183	Diverted	T	4	0	41%
16	12-FEB-03 17:52	Spont	VT	186	Diverted	T	9	0	31%
15	12-FEB-03 17:51	Spont	VT-1	180	No Thpy Pgmd	T	3	0	37%
14	12-FEB-03 17:47	Spont	VT	183	Diverted	T	5	0	28%
13	12-FEB-03 17:46	Spont	VT	186	Diverted	T	8	0	0%
12	12-FEB-03 17:44	Spont	VT-1	180	No Thpy Pgmd	T	6	0	31%
11	12-FEB-03 17:38	Spont	VT-1	183	No Thpy Pgmd	T	3	0	37%
10	12-FEB-03 17:15	Spont	VT	188	31J	T	12	0	34%
9	12-FEB-03 17:11	Spont	VT	188	31J	T	7	0	34%
8	12-FEB-03 17:06	Spont	VT	186	31J	T	3	0	34%
7	12-FEB-03 17:02	Spont	VT	194	Diverted	T	8	0	31%
6	12-FEB-03 17:00	Spont	VT	185	31J	T	8	0	34%
5	12-FEB-03 16:18	Spont	VT	182	Diverted	T	3	0	34%
4	06-FEB-03 18:09	Spont	VT-1	174	No Thpy Pgmd	T	7	0	28%
3	30-JAN-03 20:36	Spont		127	Nonsustained	F	0	0	6%
2	30-JAN-03 12:19	Spont	VT-1	171	No Thpy Pgmd	T	6	0	28%
1	27-JAN-03 21:54	Spont	VT-1	175	No Thpy Pgmd	T	11	0	12%

1 PVCs may conduct _____ to the atria and initiate an SVT.

2 The time interval between an R and P wave during typical AVNRT is _____ than that with retrograde conduction.

Addendum: About 3 months later she presented to the office for follow-up without having any complaints. The logbook from her device showed multiple episodes of ATP (anti-tachycardia ventricular burst pacing) therapy, with each one successfully converting apparent typical AVNRT.

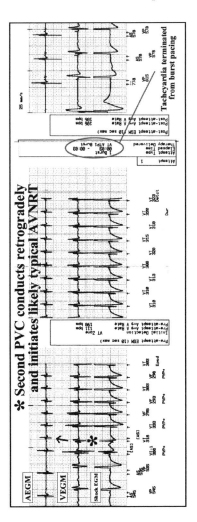

Case 24 (∗∗∗)

A 70-year-old male with ischemic cardiomyopathy (EF 20%) and complete heart block was upgraded from a dual-chamber pacemaker to ICD due to inducible VT (225 b.p.m.). He comes into the office for evaluation after receiving his first shock. The ICD is programmed as a single-zone device, VF ≥ 185 b.p.m. (all 31 J shocks), and is not committed. You interrogate the ICD and find the following recorded event.

Q Why did he receive a shock?

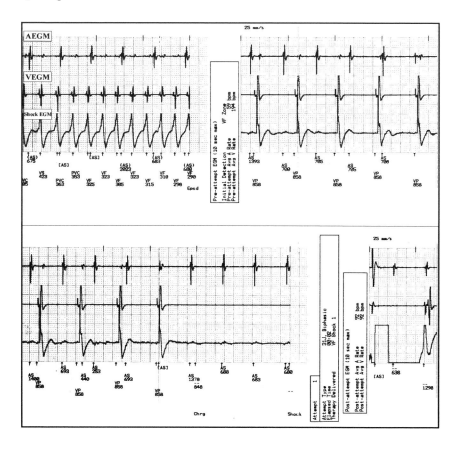

A No sensed ventricular events following charging

The tachycardia is clearly VT, and terminates spontaneously as the device begins to charge. After completion of charging, this model ICD (Guidant Prizm) makes a determination of the need to divert the shock due to a non-sustained rhythm. In order for a divert to occur in this ICD model, however, "slow" (below rate cutoff) ventricular events need to be sensed. Paced beats are not counted as slow in this device. Because there were no sensed ventricular events, due to the patient's complete heart block, the ICD assumes the rhythm to be VF too fine to be sensed and delivers a shock.

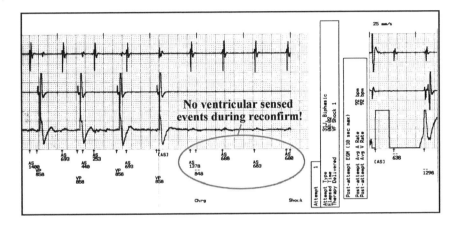

The mechanism by which ICD shocks are diverted due to non-sustained arrhythmias may slightly differ, depending on the ICD manufacturer, and the generation of the ICD. It is suggested that one consults the physician's manual of the particular model in question to see how this may occur.

Management Solution: None necessarily needed. Should this event repeat itself an upgrade to a newer generation Guidant ICD or another manufacturer's ICD whose algorithms have eliminated this phenomenon may be considered. The use of medications to help suppress frequent non-sustained VT is another consideration.

1 Different ICD models have _____ algorithms for determining whether a shock needs to be diverted.

2 A _____ VT can result in an ICD shock.

Case 25 (**)

A 55-year-old male with ischemic cardiomyopathy (EF 15%) and ICD with a dual ventricular coil implanted for a primary VF arrest is admitted for evaluation following a syncopal episode. Evaluation does not reveal any suggestion of myocardial infarction or change in cardiac function. You interrogate the ICD and obtain the following event recording. All shock impedances are normal. After questioning the patient it is learned that his general cardiologist had initiated amiodarone 3 months ago for AF. The DFT at implant was 18 J.

Q What likely happened?

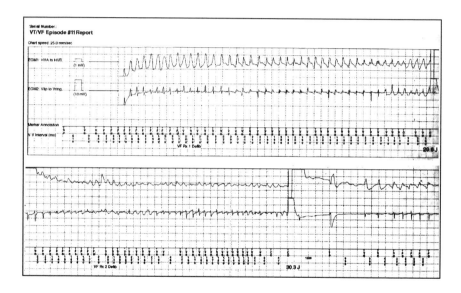

A Increased DFT from amiodarone

The first shock did not convert VF at maximum energy output! Enough time passed before the rhythm was successfully converted to cause hemo-dynamic collapse and syncope.

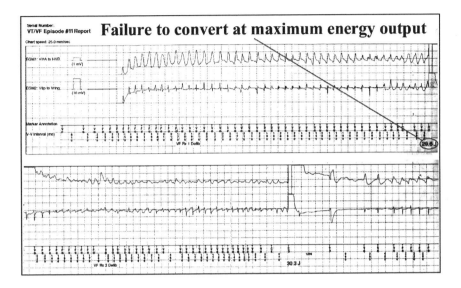

Amiodarone can significantly elevate the DFT and likely did so in this case. Other AADs also share this potential. As such a determination of DFT may be required once initial loading has completed.

Management Solution: (i) Consider discontinuing amiodarone. (ii) Consider initiating sotalol which may lower DFT. (iii) Consider reversing shock polarity and retesting. (iv) Consider upgrading the ICD to a high-energy device that would allow an appropriate shock safety margin vs. adding a subcutaneous patch/array. (v) Educate the general cardiologist as to the potential adverse effects of AADs on ICD function.

1 _____ may have significant interactions with ICD function.

2 Failure of an ICD to convert _____ at maximum output requires intervention to provide an acceptable safety margin.

Case 26 (∗∗∗)

A 67-year-old male with a right pectoral dual chamber pacemaker is undergoing implant of a left pectoral ICD due to inducible VT. Prior to induction of VF the pacemaker is programmed DOO with pacing outputs set to 7.5 V.

Q What happened during the ICD testing below?

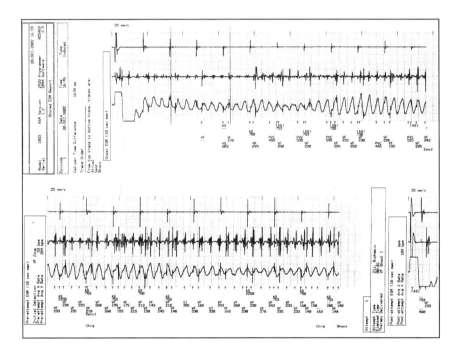

A Significant pacemaker ICD interaction

The pacemaker spikes caused significant undersensing and delayed recognition of the VF. In fact it took almost 16 seconds from the time of induction until the 21 J shock was delivered.

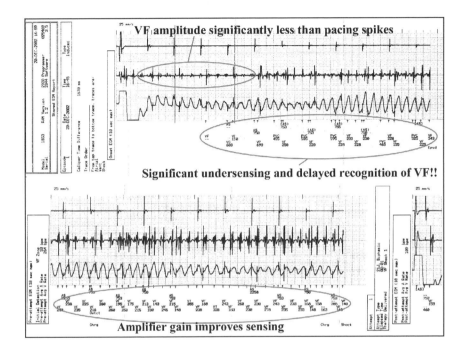

This interaction represents one of the most significant pacemaker/ICD interactions. The worst, however, is the complete lack of recognition of VF, which could be very deadly!

Management Solution: Remove pacemaker generator. It is not simply enough to program pacemaker outputs down because the pacemaker could potentially revert to a noise mode when exposed to such things as an ICD shock. In noise mode the pacemaker outputs are typically high.

1 _____ _____ is used to determine significant ICD/pacemaker interplay.

2 ICD/pacemaker interactions can be _____.

Case 27 (****)

A 71-year-old male with a dual chamber ICD implanted for VT 3 years ago is admitted following multiple shocks without warning. You interrogate the ICD and note multiple shock episodes and diverted/non-sustained episodes similar in appearance to the "rhythm" below (AEGM, VEGM, and shock EGM from top to bottom). The atrial lead impedance is 243 Ω (631 Ω at implant) and the ventricular lead impedance is 560 Ω (700 Ω at implant). You are able to reproduce the "rhythm" by having the patient cough and move the left arm.

Q What is likely happening?

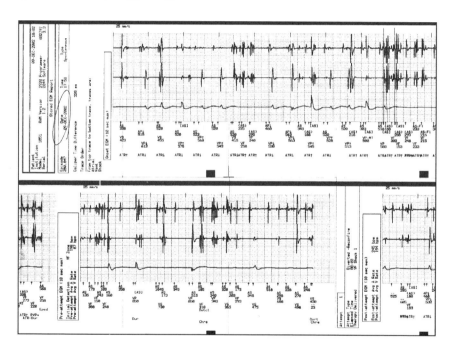

A Atrial and ventricular lead insulation defects

The most obvious finding on the strip is "noise" on both the AEGM and VEGM, but not on the shock EGM. The noise is initiating mode switching and sensing in the ICD VF zone. In fact the noise patterns on the AEGM and VEGM look nearly identical. This finding suggests that the atrial and ventricular pacing/sensing channels are intermittently in direct electrical communication. The suspected cause was dual insulation defects of the leads at their insertion site in the subclavian vein, between the first rib and clavicle, that allowed "make and break" potentials between both leads (remember that lead impedances may drop with insulation defects). These defects were not obvious under radiologic examination, but subsequently confirmed during system revision.

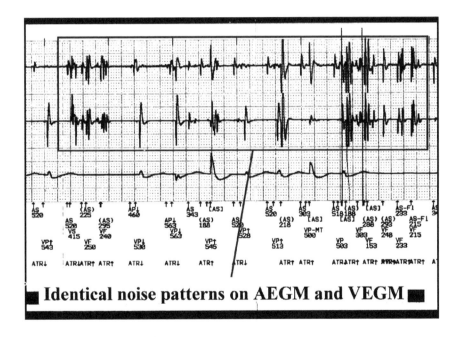

Management Solution: Prior to inpatient lead revision, turn off all VT/VF detection so as to avoid inappropriate shocks until definitive surgical management is complete.

1 A significant _____ in lead impedance can suggest an insulation defect.

2 Noise signals sensed on the atrial and ventricular channels may _____ pacing, initiate _____ switching, and cause inappropriate _____.

Case 28 (**)

A 47-year-old female has a dual chamber ICD with atrial anti-tachyarrhythmia therapies programmed on.

Q What is seen below?

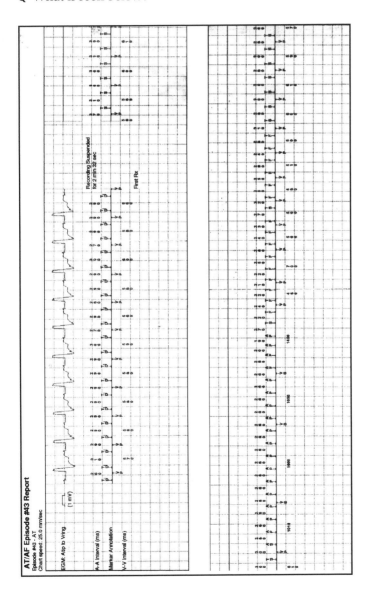

A Detection of atrial tachycardia with failure of overdrive burst pacing to terminate

The single EGM is measured between the atrial and ventricular lead tips. This displays both an atrial and ventricular EGM component, and allows one to see an atrial tachycardia conducting 2 : 1 to the ventricles. The EGM recording ceases (normal device function per the manufacturer), but the marker channels show a single round of atrial burst overdrive pacing that fails to terminate the arrhythmia (in fact it temporarily speeds it up).

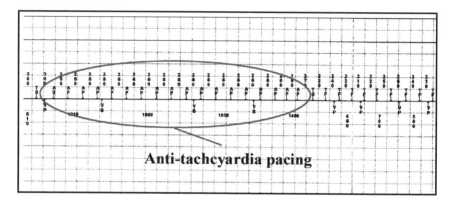

Overdrive burst pacing, as well as high frequency pacing (i.e. 50 Hz) in the atria have been utilized for treatment of atrial tachycardia and AF, respectively. Low energy shocks have also been used with some success.

Management Solution: Consider more aggressive atrial anti-tachycardia functions, including cardioversion. This needs to be weighed against the frequency of the arrhythmia, and the ability of the patient to tolerate shocks for it. AAD use and catheter ablation are also potential adjunctive resources.

1 An EGM may be recorded in some ICDs that _____ both atrial and ventricular activity.

2 Some ICD models have additional treatment options for atrial _____ and _____.

Case 29 (***)

An 82-year-old male with a history of ICD for "almost 20 years" for survived cardiac arrest is referred from an outside hospital. You obtain the following image under fluoroscopy.

Q Identify the hardware by matching the following choices with the letters on the image:

1. 5-French atrial pacemaker lead
2. 7-French atrial pacemaker lead
3. Coronary sinus left ventricular lead
4. Endocardial rate/sensing lead
5. Epicardial defibrillator patch
6. Right ventricular defibrillator lead
7. Screw-in right ventricular pacemaker lead
8. Surface ECG lead
9. Tined right ventricular rate-sensing lead

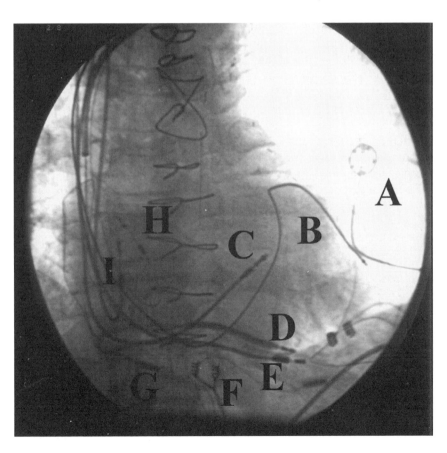

A The following letters match the following hardware:

H 1. 5-French atrial pacemaker lead
I 2. 7-French atrial pacemaker lead
B 3. Coronary sinus left ventricular lead
F 4. Endocardial rate/sensing lead
G 5. Epicardial defibrillator patch
D 6. Right ventricular defibrillator lead
C 7. Screw-in right ventricular pacemaker lead
A 8. Surface ECG lead
E 9. Tined right ventricular rate-sensing lead

One can essentially trace the natural history/evolution of the ICD through this one image alone! First, the patient received an abdominal ICD with epicardial patches and endocardial rate/sensing leads. The rate/sensing leads were prone to fracture, so an endovascular right ventricular tined rate/sensing lead was inserted and tunneled from the chest to the pocket in the abdomen. Bradyarrhythmias developed, so a right pectoral dual chamber pacemaker was implanted. Finally, medically refractory CHF symptoms ensued and a left pectoral biventricular ICD was placed, with removal of the abdominal and right pectoral generators.

Obviously the amount of hardware placed here is generous. The patient is at risk for "superior vena cava syndrome" (SVC syndrome) (obstruction of the SVC with resultant swelling of the head/neck and upper extremities) due to the large number of leads in the vascular tree. One might have contemplated a laser extraction of some of the leads with the implant of the biventricular system.

The presence of the epicardial patches can also be potentially problematic by insulating the heart from external shocks. Should an external cardioversion/defibrillation be needed, the external patches need to be placed so as to have an appropriate shocking vector (anterior–posterior in this case).

Management Solution: Follow for signs of SVC syndrome.

1 An _____ of the SVC may cause swelling of the head/neck and upper extremities.

2 Epicardial patches can _____ the heart from an external shock.

Case 30 (**)

While upgrading a patient with CHF and a single chamber pacemaker to a biventricular ICD the following image is obtained.

Q Is there anything potentially problematic with the system as implanted?

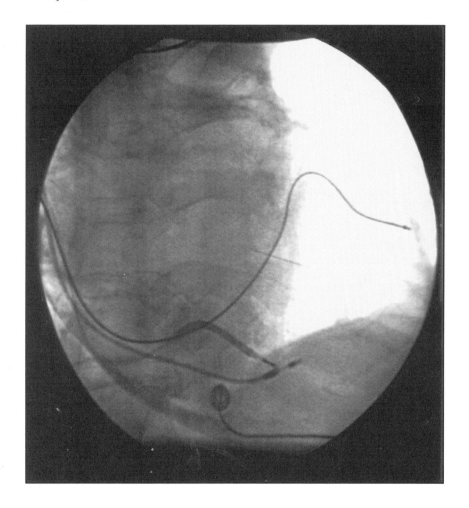

A Yes

The ICD lead tip and pacemaker lead may be touching. Also, the ICD lead tip may not be as far into the apex of the right ventricle as one would like for an optimal shocking vector.

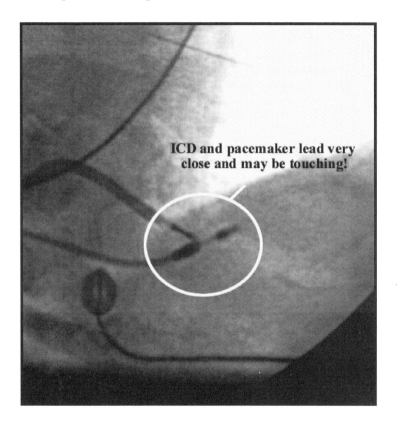

The physical contact of the pacemaker lead with the ICD lead tip can produce potentials that may be sensed and falsely interpreted by the ICD as fast ventricular events. Also, as mentioned earlier, a right ventricular ICD lead placement in the distal apex may improve the shocking vector and DFT.

Management Solution: (i) Fluoroscopically observe the leads in multiple views to confirm whether they are touching or in close proximity. Independent movement of each lead is also another indication that they are not touching/close. (ii) Consider the need to reposition the ICD lead further into the heart depending on the DFT.

1 Contact of a ventricular defibrillator and pacemaker lead near/close to their tips can produce _____ that may be sensed as _____ events.

2 A ventricular defibrillator lead tip placed at a distance away from the RV apex can result in an elevated _____.

Case 31 (*)

An 85-year-old male with a dual chamber ICD placed 4 years ago for VT is admitted for pleuritic chest pain. He also states that he has been having an "electrical" sensation in his chest for the past 2 weeks. A 12-lead ECG demonstrates changes consistent with pericarditis. Evaluation of the ICD up to this point in time has been unremarkable. ICD interrogation now shows the following lead impedances and real-time EGMs. There is no atrial pacing capture or output seen, even at maximum output.

Q What is likely wrong?

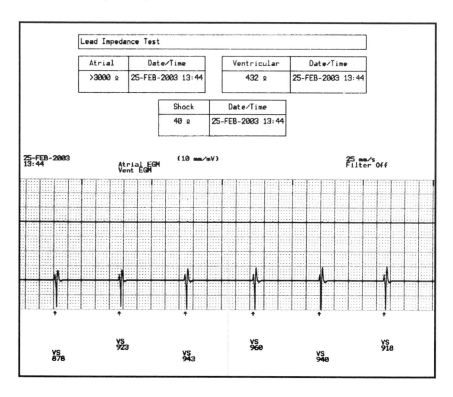

A Complete atrial lead fracture

The most noticeable features on interrogation are that the atrial lead impedance is > 3000 Ω and there is nothing recorded on the AEGM. This along with complete loss of atrial capture raised the suspicion of a complete atrial lead fracture. This was confirmed on radiologic evaluation, and demonstrated that the fractured lead end had migrated to a branch off the right main pulmonary artery (this is extremely rare)! Whether the patient's symptoms and pericarditis were a result of this was subject for speculation, but not deemed unreasonable at the time.

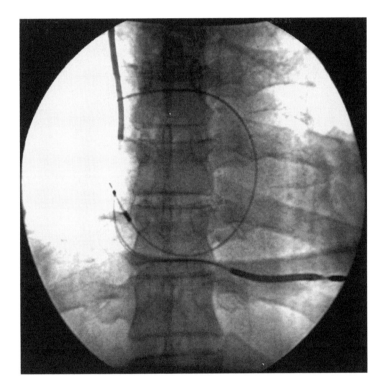

As with pacemaker leads, the leads of an ICD system can fracture at the first rib and clavicle due to crush injury between the two bones, especially when inserted by a subclavian vein puncture, in my experience.

Management Solution: (i) Implant new atrial lead (consider via an axillary vein or cephalic vein approach*) and remove old atrial lead. Removal of the old atrial lead was accomplished by introducing a snare and deflectable catheter inserted in the right femoral vein. This allowed the lead end to be pulled into the inferior vena cava, unscrewing of the lead tip, and removal through the femoral vein. (ii) Follow ventricular lead closely for any signs of compromised integrity.

1 An _____ lead impedance can suggest that a lead is fractured.

2 The _____ rib and _____ may crush a lead between them and result in significant damage over time.

---

* The axillary vein can be accessed lateral to the junction of the first rib and clavicle. The cephalic vein can be accessed by a "cut-down" approach in the delto-pectoral groove. Some physicians believe both of these avenues of venous entry may be less likely to fracture due to trauma between the first rib and clavicle.

Case 32 (**)

Prior to closing the pocket of a newly implanted dual chamber ICD interrogation of the system is performed with a sterile wand.

Q What is the problem?

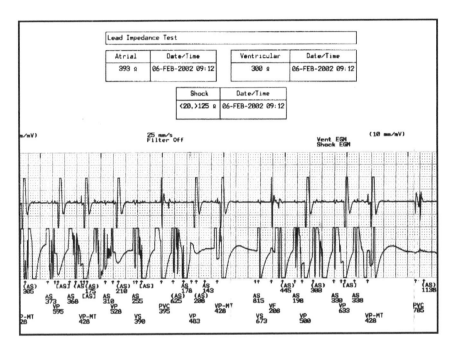

A Loose shock set screw

The shock impedance is out of range and there is noise on the shock EGM. A loose shock set screw in the ICD header was demonstrated on re-inspection of the ventricular lead.

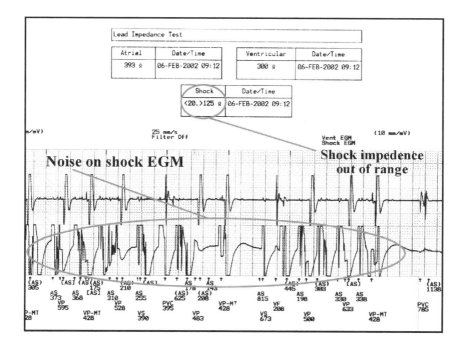

A loose shock set screw could result in the inability to defibrillate! Meticulous care to insert each system component in the header with visualization of the lead pins past the set screw, and then applying an appropriate number of turns to place the set screw should avoid this sort of situation.

Management Solution: Tighten shock set screw.

1 A loose set screw in the _____ and _____ ports, respectively, can cause inappropriate shocks and an inability to successfully cardiovert/defibrillate.

2 Loose set screws can generally be avoided with meticulous care to _____ them appropriately.

Case 33 (**)

Five months after undergoing placement of a dual chamber ICD for inducible VT a 43-year-old female is admitted after receiving multiple shocks without warning. The weekly average lead impedances, as measured by the device, and a non-sustained "tachycardia" episode, recorded by the ICD, are seen below.

Q What are the two likely candidates in the differential diagnosis of this problem?

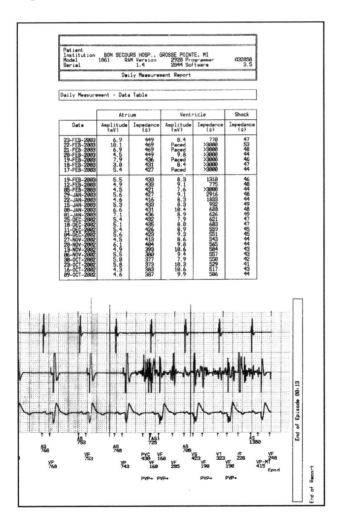

A Loose ventricular rate/sensing set screw vs. ventriuclar lead fracture

The weekly ventricular lead rate/sensing impedances have frequently become quite elevated, and there is noise seen on the VEGM. Possible likely causes include a set screw that loosened over time, and a fracture of the rate/sensing portion of the ventricular lead. A fracture occurring this early after implant would be unusual. This is not unheard of, and has been seen in my experience when the operator used a subclavian vein approach for implantation. A mechanical defect in the ICD generator itself that developed over time and caused such findings has never been seen in my experience. In this patient, however, neither of the two likely considerations could be definitively demonstrated.

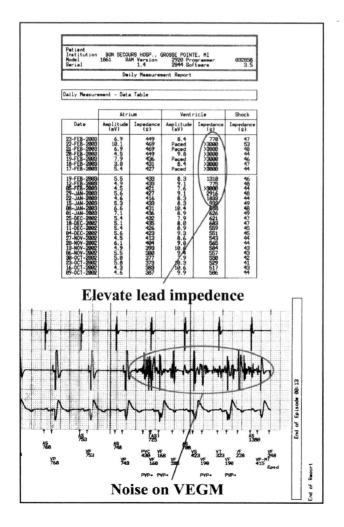

As this case demonstrates the exact cause of a problem may not be comfortably diagnosed.

Management Solution: Given the inability to adequately define the likely problem, a new ventricular lead was implanted (via an axillary vein approach), the set screws placed with meticulous care after plugging into the ICD, and the old ventricular lead removed.

Case 34 (**)

A 59-year-old male with an ICD is undergoing neck surgery. The ICD fires, shortly after the first burst from an electric cautery knife. The surgeon explains that he has always used short bursts of cautery before and never had any issues with an ICD. He calls the ICD manufacturer's representative to the procedure to find out why this happened.

Q What might they have found?

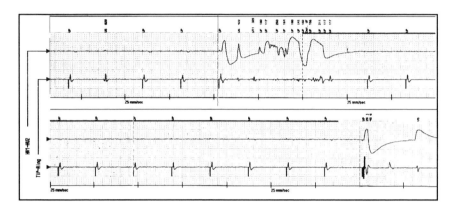

A ICD programmed with committed therapy

Unbeknownst to the surgeon, the ICD was programmed committed to shock once detection criterion was satisfied. Detection was quickly satisfied with even this short burst of cautery, which initiated capacitor charging, and then the subsequent committed shock.

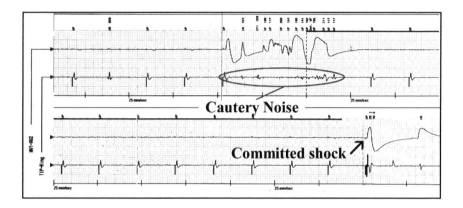

As mentioned earlier, the "noise" generated by an electric cautery knife may be easily sensed as ventricular activity by an ICD. Short bursts from the knife, while being sensed, do not typically result in a shock, unless, as in the rare case above, the device is programmed to be committed once detection has been satisfied. Such an episode can always be avoided by turning off detection and/or therapies before cautery is used.

Management Solution: ALWAYS interrogate an ICD and ensure that detection and/or therapies are programmed off prior to the planned use of an electric cautery knife.

1 An ICD programmed for _____ therapy will treat a non-sustained event that satisfies detection criterion.

Case 35 (****)

DFT testing is being performed during implantation of a dual chamber ICD at least ventricular sensitivity for the device.

Q Why did it take so long to shock the rhythm?

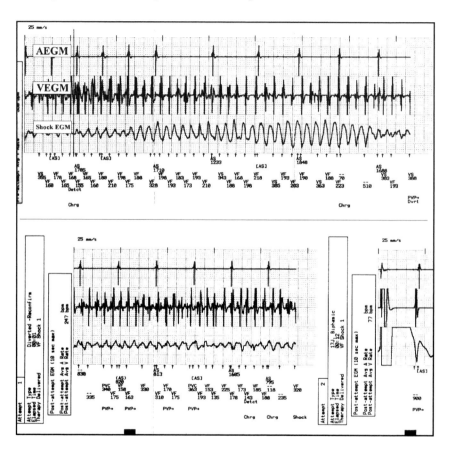

A Ventricular undersensing causing a shock diversion

The least sensitive setting caused numerous ventricular "drop-out" beats (undersensed beats) to occur. At the end of the upper strip the ICD found enough "slow" ventricular beats (below rate cutoff), due to drop-out, to think that the arrhythmia had terminated. Thus it diverted the shock.

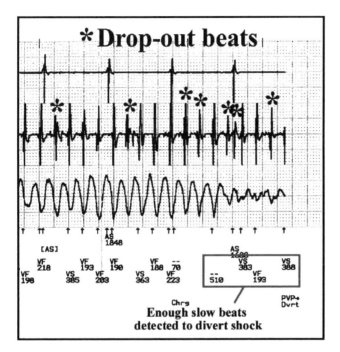

It has been found most useful in my experience to test an ICD at implant with a least sensitive setting. If there is no undersensing during this maneuver, then one knows that sensitivity can be safely adjusted in the future from a nominal setting to a less sensitive setting without the need for additional VF testing (i.e. as one might do in an outpatient arena for such things as T wave oversensing). In the above situation, this is not the case.

Management Solution: Maintain adequate sensitivity such that undersensing is less likely to occur and delay/prevent appropriate timely treatment.

1 A _____ ventricular sensitivity can result in signal drop-out during VF detection.

2 T wave _____ may be compensated for by decreasing ventricular sensitivity.

Case 36 (★★★★)

Two weeks after implantation of a biventricular ICD for CHF a 53-year-old male returns to the hospital after receiving a shock without warning. The ICD is programmed with a single zone of therapy, VF ≥ 185 b.p.m. (23 J followed by all 31 J shock), and ventricular sensitivity at nominal. The pacing mode is DDD with a lower rate 40 b.p.m., AV interval 90 ms, and upper rate 150 b.p.m. The EGM sequence leading to the shock is seen below.

Q What happened?

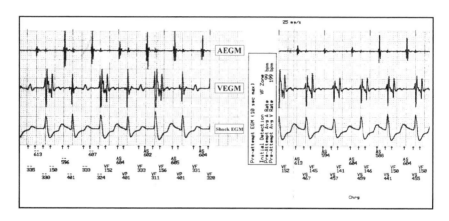

A T wave oversensing facilitates QRS double counting

The T waves with ventricular pacing are oversensed. Each time this occurs the subsequent P wave is sensed, but ventricular pacing not delivered 90 ms following (AV interval) as this violates the upper rate. The native ventricular QRS complexes are double counted. The ICD then thinks it has detected an arrhythmia and changes the pacing mode to a back-up of VVI. This then allows continuous double counting of each QRS complex and the subsequent shock.

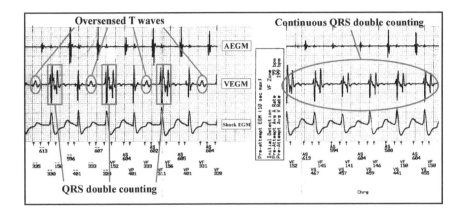

As discussed earlier, some biventricular ICDs utilize both right and left ventricular lead sensing for tachyarrhythmia detection. The mechanism facilitating the double counting here, as opposed to earlier cases, was different.

Management Solution: (i) Decrease ventricular sensitivity to a setting that eliminates T wave oversensing, but does not produce undersensing of VF. (ii) If double counting remains an issue despite elimination of T wave oversensing then consider changing the ICD generator to one that does not utilize left ventricular sensing for tachycardia detection.

1 An ICD that does not utilize _____ ventricular sensing for tachycardia detection will not allow double counting from two separate ventricular leads each sensing the same event.

Case 37 (∗∗∗)

A patient with a biventricular ICD and pre-existing LBBB is undergoing a ventricular pacing threshold test. The mode is DDD with a lower rate of 40 b.p.m. and an AV interval of 80 ms.

Q Identify the points on the strips where LV and RV capture are lost.

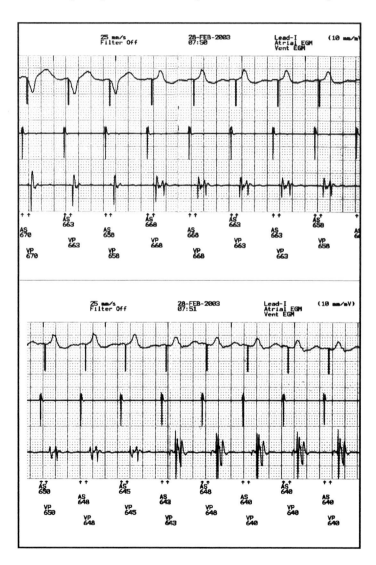

A The points where LV and RV capture are lost are shown below:

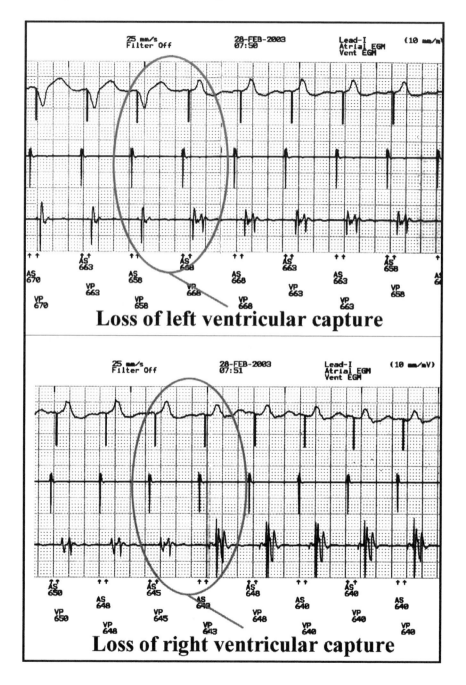

Surface ECG lead I in addition to the VEGM has been most useful in my experience for assisting in the determination of ventricular pacing thresholds in a biventricular ICD without separate left and right ventricular pacing programmability. Biventricular pacing capture in surface lead I typically has a negative QRS complex. The transition to a positive QRS complex in lead I signifies the onset of a LBBB, and thus loss of at least LV capture in this patient. The transition to loss of RV capture here is subtle on the surface lead as the progression is from a pacing induced to a native LBBB. What is not so subtle here is the change in R wave morphology on the VEGM that greatly aids in the identification of this transition.

1 Biventricular pacing commonly causes a predominantly _____ QRS complex in surface lead I.

2 ECG changes on single surface leads during biventricular pacing threshold testing can be very _____.

Case 38 (***)

A 65-year-old male with a dual chamber ICD (not biventricular) placed for VT at an outside hospital comes into the ER having had multiple shocks in succession. A representative example of the events recorded by the ICD is seen below. Chest radiography displays appropriate positioning of both atrial and ventricular leads.

Q What happened?

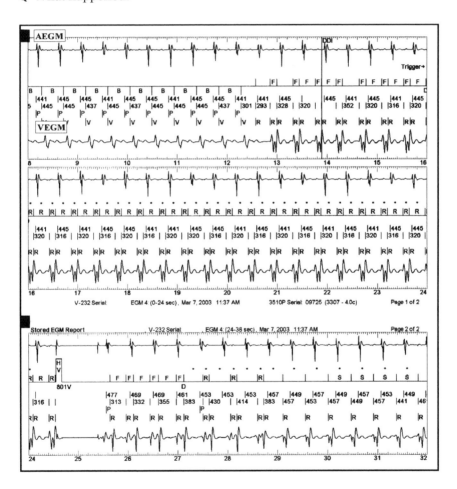

A T wave oversensing facilitates QRS double counting

The initial rhythm is P wave tracking. Next, a T wave is oversensed. Ventricular pacing does not then occur, as this would have violated the upper tracking limit. This results in double counting of each QRS, detection in the VF zone, and finally a high energy shock.

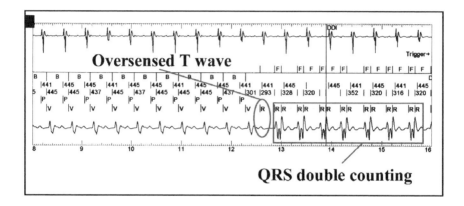

It is unusual to see QRS double counting by a single ventricular ICD lead. It was theorized that this patient's native bundle branch block was severe enough, and the far-field signal from the delayed ventricle large enough to result in the double counting.

Management Solution: A parameter specific to this manufacturer's device, the "decay delay" was altered so as to eliminate the native QRS double counting. Also, decreased ventricular sensitivity to eliminate T wave over-sensing, without compromising VF detection, was programmed.

1 QRS double counting _____ occur in both a biventricular and a standard ICD.

Case 39 (**)

The evening after undergoing placement of a biventricular ICD (integrated bipolar right ventricular lead) for Class IV CHF, a 57-year-old male is noted to have an intermittent change in the appearance of his QRS complex on telemetry. Thresholds of the left ventricular coronary sinus and right ventricular leads at implant were 1.7 and 0.6 V, respectively, at 0.5 ms. There was no evidence of RV anodal capture at high output. You interrogate the ICD and print the following rhythm strip at 7.5 V/2.0 ms ventricular output. The mode is DDD, lower rate 40 b.p.m., and AV interval 80 ms. You suspect something is wrong and make arrangements to bring him back to the electrophysiology laboratory the next morning.

Q What was your suspicion?

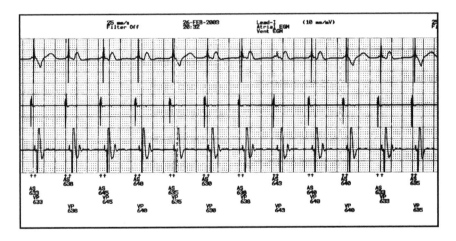

A Dislodged left ventricular lead

There is intermittent left ventricular capture noted on the rhythm strip (see Case 37 for further explanation). Given this, it was suspected that the left ventricular lead had become slightly dislodged. In fact, by the next morning the left ventricular lead was noted to be completely dislodged out of the coronary sinus anatomy.

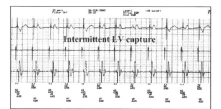

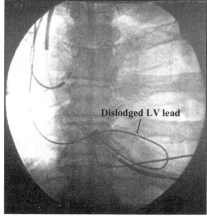

The current model of left ventricular coronary sinus lead has tines to help lodge itself in a coronary sinus vein. Even as such they only rarely dislodge in experienced hands. This particular lead had originally been placed in a lateral coronary sinus branch.

Management Solution: Reposition left ventricular lead in a stable position.

1 Contemporary LV coronary sinus pacing leads are a type of _____ fixation lead.

2 _____ of an LV coronary sinus pacing lead is rare in experienced hands.

Case 40 (*)

A 63-year-old federal court judge, with no prior arrhythmia or syncope history, requires a biventricular ICD for Class III CHF, with the left ventricular lead via an epicardial route. He wishes only initially to have the basic ICD implant, after which he will clear his schedule and return for the epicardial lead. Two weeks prior to the scheduled epicardial lead placement you are called to interrogate his ICD in a local ER trauma ward. Apparently while driving, the patient passed out and struck a tree, amazingly without significant injury. His potassium is found to be 2.1 mEq/dL. The EGMs leading to an appropriate successful shock are seen below.

Q What happened?

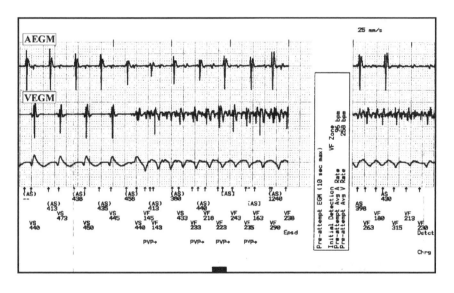

A Hypokalemia-induced VF

The patient had spontaneous VF that likely caused syncope prior to successful conversion.

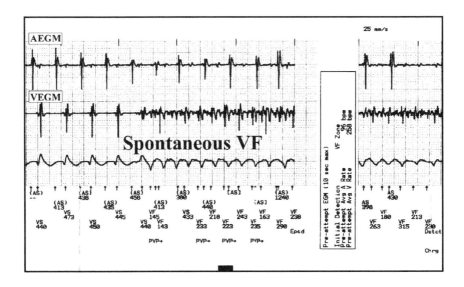

It is not uncommon to see significant ventricular tachyarrhythmias in the setting of hypokalemia. This situation does not necessarily require the institution of an antiarrhythmic medicine (i.e. amiodarone).

Management Solution: Correct the electrolyte abnormality with careful vigilance to maintain subsequent potassium levels in an appropriate range. As regards the use of a motor vehicle by a patient with an ICD, the laws vary depending on the patient's state of residence.

1 _____ can cause significant ventricular tachyarrhythmias.

2 Despite an expedient detection and termination of VF, a patient may have _____ during the event.

Case 41 (**)

A 65-year-old male presents to the ER after having received "many" shocks in the setting of palpitations. The patient's arrhythmia logbook confirms his complaint.

Q What may have happened?

```
┌─────────────────────────────────────────────────────────────────────┐
│ ┌───────────────────────────────────────────────────────────────┐   │
│ │                                                                 │   │
│ │ Patient                              01-MAY-2003 07:25          │   │
│ │ Institution                                                     │   │
│ │ Model      1861    RAM Version   2920 Programmer      030296    │   │
│ │ Serial             1.4           2844 Software           3.5    │   │
│ ├───────────────────────────────────────────────────────────────┤   │
│ │            Arrhythmia Logbook Report                            │   │
│ └───────────────────────────────────────────────────────────────┘   │
```

Episode Query Selections

Show All Episodes

Episode	Date/Time	Type	Zone	Rate bpm	Therapy/Duration	V>A	Stab ms	AFib	Ons
14	26-APR-03 03:44	Spont	VF	212	21J,31J,31Jx	T	13	0	41%
13	26-APR-03 03:42	Spont	VF	211	21J	T	5	0	22%
12	26-APR-03 03:41	Spont	VF	211	21J	T	5	0	19%
11	26-APR-03 03:39	Spont	VF	207	21J	T	6	0	22%
10	26-APR-03 03:37	Spont	VF	206	21J	T	22	0	28%
9	26-APR-03 03:35	Spont	VF	212	21J	T	9	0	19%
8	26-APR-03 03:27	Spont		132	Nonsustained	F	N/R	0	25%
7	26-APR-03 03:24	Spont	VF	211	21J	T	11	0	25%
6	26-APR-03 03:10	Spont	VF	211	21J	T	10	0	28%
5	26-APR-03 03:06	Spont	VF	203	Diverted	T	8	0	25%
4	26-APR-03 02:40	Spont	VF	190	21J	T	28	0	47%
3	26-APR-03 02:00	Spont	VF	194	21J	T	5	0	37%
2	26-APR-03 01:35	Spont	VF	183	21J	T	4	0	34%
1	25-APR-03 23:55	Spont	VF	189	21J,31J	T	7	0	28%

A System malfunction vs. shocks for SVT vs. shock for frequent VT/VF

Whenever a patient receives multiple shocks a malfunction of the system needs to be considered. For example a loose set screw or ventricular lead fracture causing "make and break" potentials could cause such a situation. External electromagnetic interference, generous myopotential oversensing, or T wave oversensing could also cause unexpected and frequent shocks. Second, an SVT with rapid ventricular response may fall into the ICD treatment zone and may persist despite a shock. Finally, frequent and recurrent VT/VF can occur in the setting of an electrolyte abnormality, cardiac ischemia, or a medication change (i.e. anti-arrhythmic drug). It can also occur de novo. Here the patient had de novo VT that frequently recurred. This is a situation sometimes referred to as "VT storm" (see continuous excerpt below).

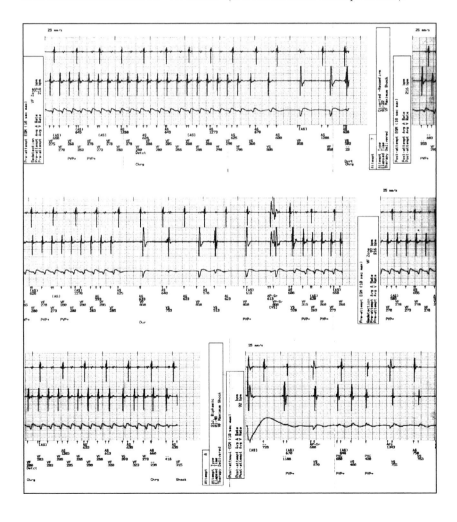

Management Solution: Consider long-term AAD use vs. VT ablation.

1 _____ storm may cause multiple shocks within a very short period of time.

2 A patient receiving an appropriate shock after the onset of significant chest pain may have VT/VF in the setting of cardiac _____.

Case 42 (*)

The following EGMs are noted during VF induction in a 51-year-old female undergoing DFT testing.

Q What happened here?

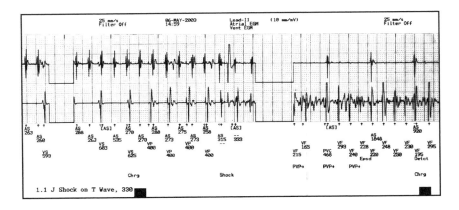

A Atrial tachycardia terminated, VF induced

VF was induced with the 1.1 J shock on T wave. The shock also terminated the atrial tachycardia.

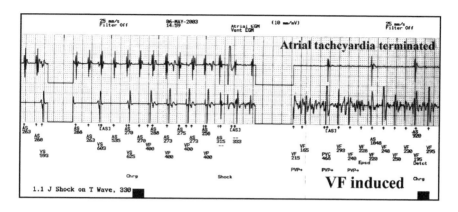

Atrial tachyarrhythmias, including AF/flutter, may not uncommonly be terminated during DFT testing, either during the induction shock, or during the defibrillation shock. For patients with persistent or chronic AF/flutter it is important to know whether they have been appropriately treated with anti-coagulation or have no atrial clot on trans-esophageal echocardiography prior to DFT testing. This is because termination of AF/flutter could precipitate a thrombo-embolic event were a clot to be present.

Management Solution: Confirm appropriate anti-coagulation, or absence of cardiac thrombus, in patients with AF/flutter prior to DFT testing.

1 An ICD shock can both terminate and _____ an arrhythmia.

2 One method of _____ induction is a "shock-on-T."

Case 43 (****)

An 80-year-old male with chronic AF and a right pectoral dual chamber permanent pacemaker has just had a biventricular ICD (atrial port plugged) implanted at the left pectoral region. Prior to its removal the pacemaker is reprogrammed to a DDI mode after therapies in the ICD are disabled. The ICD pacing mode is VVI at 40 b.p.m.

Q Is there anything unusual about the following rhythm strip recorded during this time?

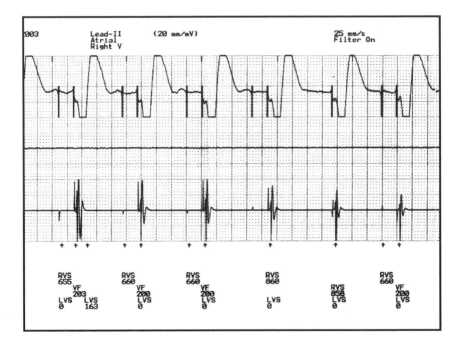

A Yes

First, the patient's AF is undersensed by the pacemaker as evidenced by the presence of atrial pacing. The first, second, third, and sixth atrial pacing spikes from the permanent pacemaker are oversensed as ventricular events by the ICD. This causes each of the subsequent paced QRS complexes from the pacemaker to fall into the ICD's VF detection zone. The first QRS is also double detected (sensed by the RV and LV leads at a different time).

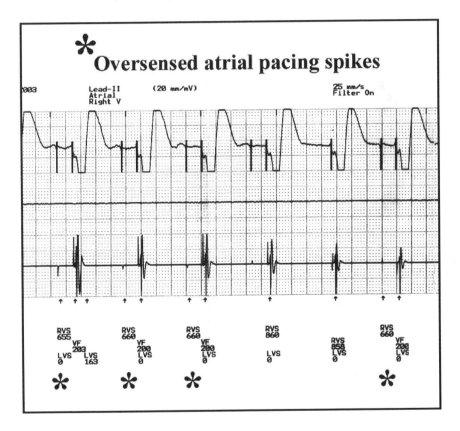

This phenomenon represents one of the other significant pacemaker/ICD interactions that can occur besides undersensing of VF. In fact if the atrial and ventricular pacing spikes are sensed at a fast enough rate the ICD can detect what it thinks is a tachyarrhythmia and deliver treatment.

Management Solution: Remove pacemaker to avoid any potential ICD/pacer interaction.

1 The pacing spikes from a separate pacemaker may be _____ by an ICD.

2 Pacemaker spikes oversensed by an ICD can be _____ in a tachycardia zone.

SECTION III

Answers

Chapter 1: What is an ICD?
1 ICD
2 SCD
3 Ventricular, Dual, Bi
4 Congestive heart failure

Chapter 2: ICD System and Cardiac Anatomy
1 Apex
2 Doesn't
3 Right atrium
4 Phrenic nerve
5 Variable

Chapter 3: The Hardware
1 4–7
2 Capacitor
3 Header
4 Can
5 Pacing/sensing, Shock
6 Can, Coil
7 1,2
8 3,2
9 Integrated, True
10 Ring
11 SVC
12 Array, Patch
13 Proximal
14 Same
15 Automatically
16 Pacing, Tachyarrhythmia
17 Annotations
18 Differ
19 EGMs
20 Event
21 Interrogating
22 Induced
23 Shock, T
24 Extra
25 Sedation, Defibrillator

Chapter 4: ICD Electronics
1 Pacing/sensing, Cardioversion/defibrillation
2 ICD
3 Inhibit, Input
4 200, 1000
5 Voltage, Charge
6 Seconds
7 Time
8 Voltage
9 25, 100
10 Fracture
11 One
12 Biphasic
13 Maximized
14 Hot can, Active can
15 Dose, Response
16 10 J
17 SVC
18 Lower
19 Can
20 Array, Patch
21 High

Chapter 5: Sensing
1 Tenths
2 T
3 Auto adjusting, Gain
4 Same

Chapter 6: Detection
1 Heart rate
2 One, Three
3 Therapy
4 Differ
5 Classified
6 Zones
7 Different
8 Any, Detected
9 Consecutive, VT

Chapter 9: ICD Pacing

1 VVI, slow
2 Precipitate
3 Remove
4 Mode, Rate
5 VDD, DDD, Slow
6 100%
7 Short, Generous
8 VVIR
9 Double counting
10 Native
11 Y
12 Newer, Left
13 Difficult
14 LBBB
15 VEGM
16 Positive
17 Negative
18 Positive
19 Three
20 Anodal, LV tip–RV ring
21 Third
22 Second

Chapter 10: Unusual ICD Situations and Alternate Applications

1 Significant
2 VF
3 Lead chatter
4 Separated
5 Sensed
6 Detection, Therapies
7 Different
8 Turn off
9 Increased, Decreased
10 Slow
11 Pacing, Cardioversion
12 CHF
13 Biventricular pacing

Chapter 12: Case Studies Part B

Case 1

1 Atrial, Pre-empted

2 Biventricular, Bundle branch block

Case 2

1 Less

2 Decreasing

Case 3

1 Sinus tachycardia

2 Sudden onset

Case 4

1 10 J

2 Dose response

Case 5

1 Below

2 Similar

Case 6

1 Simultaneously

2 TIT

Case 7

1 AF

2 Stability

Case 8

1 Double count

2 Slow

Case 9

1 T, Ventricular

2 Inappropriate

Case 10

1 Ventricular burst pacing

2 Accelerate

Case 11

1 EMI, Skeletal muscle potentials

2 Avoid

Case 12
1 Biventricular pacing, Atrial, Ventricular

Case 13
1 VT, SVT

Case 14
1 SVT
2 Supraventricular

Case 15
1 Undersensing
2 Obsolete (unnecessary)

Case 16
1 Make and break, Inhibit, Shocks
2 Loose

Case 17
1 Sensed
2 Detection, Therapies

Case 18
1 Simultaneous
2 AVNRT, Entrainment

Case 19
1 AF
2 Undersensing

Case 20
1 Supraventricular
2 Orientation

Case 21
1 High
2 Crosstalk

Case 22
1 Below
2 Faster

Case 23
1 Retrogradely
2 Shorter

Case 24
1 Different
2 Non-sustained

Case 25
1 AADs
2 VF

Case 26
1 Interaction testing
2 Deadly

Case 27
1 Decrease
2 Inhibit, Mode, Shocks

Case 28
1 Displays
2 Fibrillation, Tachycardia

Case 29
1 Obstruction
2 Insulate

Case 30
1 Potentials, Ventricular
2 DFT

Case 31
1 Elevated
2 First, Clavicle

Case 32
1 Pace/Sense, Shock
2 Tighten

Case 34
1 Committed

Case 35
1 Decreased
2 Oversensing

Case 36
1 Left

Case 37
1 Negative
2 Subtle

Case 38
1 Can

Case 39
1 Passive
2 Dislodgement

Case 40
1 Hypokalemia
2 Syncope

Case 41
1 VT
2 Ischemia

Case 42
1 Induce
2 VF

Case 43
1 Oversensed
2 Detected

Index